Notes on Psychiatry

Notes on Psychiatry

I. M. Ingram
M.D., F.R.C. Psych., D.P.M.

Consultant Psychiatrist,
Southern General Hospital, Glasgow
Honorary Clinical Lecturer in Psychological Medicine,
University of Glasgow

G. C. Timbury
M.B., F.R.C.P.Ed. & Glas., F.R.C. Psych., D.P.M.

Postgraduate Dean and
Professor of Postgraduate Medical
Education, University of Glasgow

R. M. Mowbray
M.A., Ph.D.

Associate Dean,
Faculty of Community Medicine
and Behavioural Sciences,
Memorial University, St. John's, Newfoundland

FIFTH EDITION

CHURCHILL LIVINGSTONE
EDINBURGH LONDON MELBOURNE AND NEW YORK 1981

CHURCHILL LIVINGSTONE
Medical Division of Longman Group Limited

Distributed in the United States of America by Churchill
Livingstone Inc., 19 West 44th Street, New York, N.Y.
10036, and by associated companies, branches and
representatives throughout the world.

First edition 1962
Second edition 1964
Third edition 1967
Fourth edition 1976
Fifth edition 1981

ISBN 0 443 02339 5

British Library Cataloguing in Publication Data
Ingram, Ian Malcolm
    Notes on psychiatry. – 5th ed. – (Churchill
    Livingstone medical texts)
    1. Psychiatry
    I. Title   II. Timbury, Gerald Charles
    III. Mowbray, Robert Murdoch
    616,8'9   RC454   80-41412

Printed in Singapore by Huntsmen Offset Printing Pte Ltd

Preface

These notes are deliberately concise. They are suitable for revision, but as an introduction must be supplemented by lectures, clinical experience and further reading, suggestions for which are given. They were compiled for medical students at Glasgow and first appeared in 1962. Over the years they have been found useful by undergraduates and by postgraduates requiring to revise psychiatry quickly for examinations or when beginning a psychiatric post.

This fifth edition has been largely rewritten and the text much expanded to cover recent advances in the subject and the increasingly important place of psychiatry in undergraduate and postgraduate education.

Glasgow, 1981

I.M.I.
G.C.T.
R.M.M.

Contents

1

Psychopathology

In psychiatry the patient's mental state is described in a mixture of everyday and technical terms. Sometimes everyday words are used in a special or more precise sense, e.g. 'delusion', 'confusion'. The study and description of the patient's subjective experience is called psychopathology or phenomenology. It is invaluable in *understanding* the patient's experience but is not objective and does not *explain* the symptoms. To find causes we must look for explanations in genetic, metabolic and environmental factors.

Common abnormalities

1. *Disorders of perception*

   a. *Illusions.* Objects perceived are distorted and falsely interpreted, e.g. pictures in the fire, trees in the dark taking on human shape.

   b. *Hallucinations* are perceptions arising without external stimulus. They may be auditory (hearing voices when no one is speaking), visual (visions), or somatic, e.g. bodily sensations of sexual interference. They should be distinguished from pseudo-hallucinations which usually occur in hysteria and lack conviction, e.g. the patient sees things in his 'mind's eye' or with his eyes closed. *Hypnagogic or hypnopompic hallucinations* (while falling asleep or waking) are not necessarily pathological.

   c. *Déjà vu* is one of various abnormalities of imagery. The person has a strong sense of familiarity on encountering a strange place or person. Occurs in some normals and in temporal lobe epilepsy.

2. *Disorders of thinking*

It is crucial to distinguish *form* and *content* of thought, i.e. what is thought (the content) and the way in which it is thought (the form). *Formal thought disorder* refers to disorder of form, the loss of logical, rational thinking ability found in schizophrenia.

   a. *Concrete thinking:* inability to think conceptually or abstractly. Tested by interpretation of proverbs. A person with concrete thinking cannot give the general meaning of a proverb, e.g. 'A drowning man will clutch at a straw' — 'He could breathe through it'; an ingenious but concrete response.

1

b. *Dereistic thinking:* thinking determined by mood and instinct which disregards reality, e.g. wish-fulfilling day dreams.

c. *Acceleration* (pressure of thought, flight of ideas) and *retardation.* *Clang associations,* determined by sound rather than sense may occur.

d. *Perseveration:* the persistence of thoughts and actions after they have served their purpose, e.g. patient may respond to a new question or instruction by repeating his response to the previous one.

e. *Circumstantiality:* overdetailed and roundabout thinking; inability to separate the important from the trivial.

f. *Incoherence:* thinking and speech may show *fragmentation* or *contamination* (words or parts of words fused).

g. *Thought blocking:* the experience of thought processes stopping abruptly for short periods.

3. Delusions

A delusion is a belief which cannot be accepted by others of the same class, education or cultural background and which cannot be changed by logical argument or evidence against it. The hallmarks of a true delusion are the overwhelming conviction with which it is held and its incorrigibility, even when it is absurd.

a. *Secondary delusions* are psychologically understandable as arising from (secondary to) some other abnormality such as thought disorder or mood disturbance; e.g. a depressed patient may believe that he has committed an unforgivable sin, despite a relatively blameless life. The delusion is secondary to the disturbed mood.

b. *Primary or autochthonous delusions* are psychologically incomprehensible and not derived from other psychological states. They are often preceded by a feeling of 'delusional atmosphere' or 'awareness' — a feeling of impending revelation.

c. *Delusional perceptions and misinterpretations.* Things are seen or heard normally, but special significance is attached to them. *Delusional memories* also occur.

d. *Overvalued ideas:* may be confused with delusions. They are convictions which can be understood in the light of the person's background and personality: usually propagated or defended in a fanatical way.

e. *Ideas of reference:* beliefs that normal, neutral events refer specifically to the individual. Correct perception, faulty interpretation. Common in shy adolescents and paranoid states.

f. *Passivity feelings:* the experience of thoughts, emotion, behaviour being controlled by others, e.g. thought withdrawal, thought insertion.

4. *Disorders of emotion (affect)*

a. *Depression* and *elation* may be understandable or non-understandable. The central disturbance is of vitality (increased or diminished) and is often experienced both physically and mentally.

b. *Apathy:* loss or absence of feeling.

c. *Depersonalisation:* the feeling that one has lost one's feelings; a feeling of not being real.

d. *Derealisation:* the feeling that objects and people no longer seem real, that no feeling is experienced towards them.

e. *Anxiety* and *ecstasy* are other variations in mood.

5. *Compulsive phenomena*

a. *Obsessions:* contents of consciousness from which the person cannot free himself, although he recognises them to be nonsensical or groundless. He feels compelled to think them and at the same time tries to resist them.

b. *Compulsions:* acts which the person feels compelled to carry out, e.g. touching, washing, against his own resistance and with knowledge that they are senseless.

6. *Disorders of consciousness*

Between the normal states of sleep/waking and the severe abnormality of coma there are various disorders of consciousness. In most there is *clouding of consciousness* characterised by disturbed awareness of time, place and person (disorientation). *Torpor* is a state of pathological drowsiness with clouding of consciousness. *Delirium* is the term used when physical restlessness is added. In *twilight states* the patient may appear to behave normally, but has only cloudy recall on recovery. Attention is usually narrowed and situations incompletely understood. Note that *stupor* is a state of immobility and lack of response to stimuli, *without* loss of consciousness.

7. *Disorders of memory*

Four elements of memory can be disordered: grasp, retention, recall, and recognition. Immediate and long-term memory may be separately disturbed. *Amnesia* can occur in delirious states or in clear consciousness. If grasp and retention are intact and recall alone impaired an emotional cause is likely (hysterical amnesia). Head injury may produce *retrograde* amnesia. *Confabulation:* in amnesic states the patient may confabulate, i.e. invent material to fill gaps in his memory.

8. *Orientation*

The individual's self-awareness: measured for time, place and person.

2

Classification of psychiatric disorders

Normal/abnormal

Doctors often use 'normal' and 'abnormal' as synonyms for healthy and sick, and also assume that there is an all or none distinction between the two rather than a continuum from one to the other.

Psychiatric classification involves distinguishing normal from abnormal behaviour. In this context 'normal' and 'abnormal' can mean healthy and sick, but may also be used in other senses. The terms can mean good and bad (a moral interpretation of behaviour), responsible and irresponsible (a legal interpretation) or average and deviant (a statistical interpretation based on the normal distribution curve).

Some psychiatric symptoms differ sharply from the normal and almost always indicate illness, in the same way that typical anginal pain signals physical illness. Confusion, visual hallucinations, or grossly inappropriate behaviour in public, are symptoms which differ qualitatively from the normal. In milder disorders the difference from the normal may be a matter of degree and depend on context; symptoms of anxiety (sweating, tremor, palpitations) which would indicate *anxiety neurosis* if they occurred without obvious cause, would be normal immediately before an important interview or examination.

In these milder conditions (psychoneurosis and personality disorders) signs and symptoms are best regarded as deviations from average behaviour and experience. This implies a continuum from normal to abnormal. Such statistical usage is neutral; it does not imply sickness, irresponsibility, or immorality. The idiot and the genius are both extreme deviates from an average (IQ 100) on the normal distribution curve of intelligence test scores. In terms of pathology only the idiot would be recognised as sick.

Normal and abnormal behaviour must also be placed in their social, cultural and historical context. What was normal behaviour 100 years ago may seem strange today: what is acceptable in one social class may seem strange in another, and what is tolerated in one community or country may lead to hospital admission or arrest elsewhere.

4

Because the standards for normality are complex, and the abnormal is not necessarily pathological, the division between health and disease is less clear-cut in psychiatry than in other branches of medicine. It is mainly in psychiatry that patients are found who do not accept that they are unwell, or who regard themselves as sick or wicked when the doctor does not.

Classification

In general medicine most illnesses can be classified on the basis of their aetiology, pathology, or relationship to a system of the body. In some psychiatric disorders, e.g. those due to cerebral syphilis and atherosclerosis, the same applies, but in the bulk of psychiatric disorders the causes are multiple, a combination of genetic, social and environmental factors, or not precisely known. As a result most psychiatric classification is descriptive and based on observation of symptoms, signs and the natural history of the disorder. Such a classification is crude and not entirely reliable: psychiatrists have been shown to agree reliably on the broad categories of diagnosis but to be less consistent in the specific labels they attach to patients. The use of standardised interviews, rating scales and questionnaires which can be computer analysed using statistical techniques like factor and cluster analysis helps to make diagnosis more reliable in research projects (see Ch. 4). The latest international classification of diseases contain brief definitions of the psychiatric disorders; its conscientious use by doctors should improve the quality of national and international statistics.

Three broad lines of demarcation are used:

1. The main division of mental disorders is into *mental illness* and *mental handicap* (deficiency, subnormality). Mental handicap is a condition which includes intellectual deficit and has been present from birth or an early age. Mental illness implies previous health: a disorder developing or manifesting itself later in life. The division is a very old one and has been perpetuated by legislation and by the use of separate hospitals for mental illness and mental handicap. In English law psychopathy (see p. 100) is regarded as a separate category.

2. The principle division of mental illness is into *psychoneurosis* and *psychosis*. These categories correspond to lay notions of 'nerves' and 'madness'. The psychoneuroses are common conditions whose symptoms seem understandable and can be empathised with. The psychoses are illnesses in which the symptoms are less understandable, cannot be empathised with, and in which the patient often loses contact with reality. The distinction is crude, and has exceptions, but is serviceable.

3. The terms *functional* and *organic* refer to the aetiology of the disease and are used to sub-divide the psychoses. Functional psychoses are those in which function is disturbed but no pathology can be demonstrated with current methods. Diagnosis of an illness as functional should rest on finding positive psychological symptoms and not merely upon exclusion of physical findings. Organic psychoses are those in which a demonstrable or inferred lesion is present, e.g. tumours, vascular changes, infective, toxic, traumatic or congenital factors.

Nomenclature
Variations exist, and are given in brackets, all being in common use.

Psychoneuroses
Anxiety neurosis, phobic states, hysteria, obsessional neurosis, post-traumatic neurosis, depressive neurosis.

Functional psychoses
   Affective: manic-depressive psychosis (depression or mania).
   Schizophrenia: paranoid, hebephrenic, catatonic, simple.

Organic psychoses (symptomatic psychoses)
Acute (delirium), subacute (dysmnesic syndrome, subacute delirious state), chronic (dementia), atypical.

Personality disorders

Psychosomatic disorders

Mental handicap (subnormality)
Organic, subcultural.

FURTHER READING

WHO 1978 Mental disorders: glossary and guide to their classification in accordance with the ninth revision of the international classification of diseases.

3

The psychiatric interview

The student may experience difficulties in his first encounters with psychiatric patients. Some of these difficulties arise from the nature of psychiatric symptoms and signs: disorders of emotion, of thinking, or of intelligence are less easy to elicit and describe than physical signs and symptoms. The interviewer may have to overcome his own anxieties and preconceptions about the mentally ill. Lastly, the range of information which is sought about the patient and his illness is much wider than for other clinical disciplines and requires tact, time and patience to elicit.

Nevertheless, the clinical approach is fundamentally the same as in other subjects. A methodical approach leading to a formulation of the case, which details diagnosis, prognosis and treatment, is the ultimate goal of all investigation of the patient.

During his instruction each student should interview patients and their relatives if possible, record his findings and discuss them with his teachers. In no area of medicine is practical experience more necessary, and theory less helpful.

Interviewing

The psychiatric interview is used both for investigation and psychotherapy (see p. 105). For the patient, giving a detailed and frank account of his life and problems may in itself have a therapeutic effect. The interviewer must form a good relationship with the patient and at the same time study the patient and the relationship. He is a participating observer and needs to be constantly alert to what the patient is saying and how he is behaving. The techniques necessary vary with the doctor's own personality and can be learned only by constant practice with a wide range of patients combined with self scrutiny.

The student should aim to discover the pattern of the illness, the exact nature and origin of the symptoms and to place these in the setting of the patient's personality and life history. The case history is both descriptive and developmental. The interview should cover all the material in the scheme of case taking and this may require a series of interviews. The order given need not be followed rigidly in the interview but should be adhered to in recording it. It is sensible to start the interview with the patient's present complaints rather than a detailed enquiry about his or her family history. Interviewing can be directive or non-directive and the initial investigating interview should strike a balance between direct questioning and allowing the patient to tell his story in his own way. Leading questions and interruptions should be avoided but the interview should be guided by asking for particular instances rather than generalisations and by changing the trend with comments and questions.

Recording

Make full notes at the time using the patient's own words and expressions where possible. As soon as possible after the interview the notes should be expanded and written up in terms of the scheme shown. The final case record should be legible and clearly set out. It is vital to record negative information as well as positive items. The mental state should give a vivid account of the patient's behaviour at the time of the interview and a provisional formulation and diagnosis must be made. This may require revision later but is a useful discipline. In all cases it is essential to interview and obtain further details from a relative. All notes should be signed.

Scheme of case-taking

Several interviews with a patient are usually required to complete this scheme. Where only one interview is undertaken it will be necessary to abbreviate the scheme.

Case-taking is divided into:
1. History of present illness
2. Social and personal history (supplementary history to be obtained from relative if possible)
3. Physical examination
4. Psychiatric examination (mental state)
5. Further investigations
6. Formulation.

1. History of present illness

State briefly mode of referral/admission, reason for admission and patient's complaints (in his own words), and their duration. Patient's attitude to the illness and to the referral should also be noted. Also state if a relative or friend has been seen.

Give a detailed, coherent account, in chronological order, of the illness from the earliest time at which a change was noticed until the present. Give data which will permit the onset and sequence of various symptoms to be dated as accurately as possible.

2. Social history

Family history

Father: health, age, or age at time of death, and cause of death. Personality. Occupation.

Mother: health, age, or age at time of death, and cause of death. Personality. Occupation.

Siblings: enumerate in chronological order of birth with Christian names, ages, marital status, personality, occupation, state of health (miscarriages and stillbirths to be included).

Social position and general efficiency of family. Any familial diseases, alcoholism, abnormality of personality, mental disorder, epilepsy. (If unknown or none say so.) Extend this investigation beyond the immediate family, e.g. to grandparents, uncles, aunts, cousins. Note particulars which might be required for further enquiries, e.g. names of hospitals where relatives have been treated.

Home atmosphere and influence: any important events for parents or other members of the household. Emotional relationship to parents, siblings, and relatives.

Personal history

Date and place of birth: mother's condition during pregnancy. Any complications of pregnancy or delivery. Birth weight. Breast or bottle fed.

Early development: delicate or healthy baby. Precocious or retarded. Time of teething, talking, walking, toilet training.

Neurotic symptoms in childhood: night-terrors, sleep-walking, tantrums, bed-wetting, thumb-sucking, nail-biting, faddiness about food, stammering, mannerisms, anxieties (specify).

Health during childhood: infectious diseases, chorea, infantile convulsions, etc.

School: age of beginning and finishing. Standard reached. Evidence of ability or backwardness. Special abilities or disabilities. Hobbies and interests. Relationship to schoolmates and teachers. Games.

Adolescence: attitudes to family and authority. Rebelliousness. Friendships or solitary. Fantasy life.

Occupations: age of starting work. Jobs held in chronological order, with ages, dates, reasons for change. Present economic circumstances.

Ambitions. Satisfaction in work or reasons for dissatisfaction. Military service: experience, promotion, reaction to stress.

Sexual history: age at onset of puberty (menarche, shaving); reactions. Masturbation. Fantasies. Experience. Disorders and deviations. Current outlets. Contraception.

Marriage: date of marriage, age, health and personality of spouse. Length of courtship. Marital relations.

Children: chronological list of children, giving ages, names, personality and health. Attitudes to children. Have there been miscarriages?

Habits: food, sleep, alcohol, tobacco, drugs (especially analgesics, hypnotics). Specify any change in habits.

Medical history: illnesses, operations, accidents and hospital attendances, chronologically and with details.

Previous mental illness: dates, duration, symptoms of attacks: in what hospital or out-patient department. Treatment received and response to treatment. Names and addresses of hospitals and doctors.

Antisocial behaviour: any history of violence, gambling, delinquency or criminal behaviour. Convictions, fines and sentences.

Current life situation: summary of patient's domestic and work circumstances at present time. Recent stresses or emotional conflicts of any kind.

Personality before illness

Social relations: to family, to friends and workmates. Was he/she leader, follower or organiser, aggressive, submissive, adjustable, dependent, etc?

Activities and interests: groups, societies, clubs, hobbies, books, radio, T.V., cinema.

Mood: describe in terms such as cheerful, despondent, anxious, worrying. Was he/she self-deprecating, satisfied, over-confident, stable, fluctuating (with or without any reason), controlled, demonstrative.

Character: describe in terms such as timid, sensitive, suspicious, resentful, quarrelsome, irritable, impulsive, jealous, selfish, egocentric, reserved, shy, self-conscious, strict, fussy, rigid. Give examples.

Standards: moral, religious, social, economic, practical. Attitude towards self, others, health and bodily functions.

Energy and initiative: output sustained or fitful. Easily fatigued, daily rhythm, sleep habits, ability to make decisions.

Reaction to stress: level of tolerance, types of stress (frustration, loss) and response (anger, depression). Typical or excessive defence mechanisms. Personality defects revealed by stress.

3. Physical examination

Physical examination should be comprehensive and should be carried out within a day of admission. Special attention should be given to the central nervous system. Positive and negative findings should be recorded and a brief summary of abnormalities found should be given. When possible physical examination should precede assessment of the mental state, as observation of the patient's behaviour during his examination is often informative or revealing.

4. Psychiatric examination (mental state)

General behaviour: appearance, ward behaviour since admission, and attitude to hospital, nurses, doctors, other patients. Activity. Eating and sleeping.

Talk: (describe its form here, not its content.) Much or little, Spontaneous or only in answer to questions. Rate, coherence. If abnormal, give *sample of talk*.

Mood: not only happiness or sadness but irritability, perplexity, fear or anxiety. Constancy and causes of variations. Appropriate or incongruous. Attitude to future. Suicidal thoughts.

Form of thought: ability to think in abstract terms (test with proverbs and record answers) consistently and without interruption of flow. Does patient experience blocking, pressure or poverty in thinking?

Content of thought: describe in detail the content of thought, problems and preoccupations. List main worries.

Delusions and misinterpretations. Doubts about environment. Ideas of reference, persecution. Are there delusions of self-depreciation, grandiosity, guilt, hypochondriasis, poverty, etc.

Hallucinations and other disorders of perception (auditory, visual, tactile, etc.). Manner of reception, source, vividness, occurrence. Alone? At night? Feelings of unreality or changes in the self (derealisation or depersonalisation).

Obsessional phenomena: content of obsessions and extent to which they are resisted. Recognition of their absurdity. Relation to emotional state. Association with compulsive acts and rituals.

Orientation: knowledge of name, identity, place, time, date, other persons and circumstances of admission.

Memory: estimate from patient's account of history. Test for recent and remote events, recall of a list of numbers and of a name and address — immediately and after five minutes. Immediate recall of sentence, e.g. 'The one thing a nation needs in order to be rich and great is a large secure supply of wood.' Note repetitions required to learn the sentence.

Attention and concentration: easily distracted? Preoccupied? Tests: Days and months in reverse order. Serial 7's. (Subtract 7 from 100, then from 93 and so on until 2 is reached.)

General information: test according to patient's experience and education and estimate with these in mind, e.g. using current events, Prime Minister, Royal Family, capital cities and large towns, etc.

Intelligence: estimate from history and general knowledge. Note discrepancies between this estimate and the patient's educational and occupational background.

Insight and judgement: attitude to present state. Regarded as illness? In need of treatment? Plans for future. Attitude to any financial, domestic or ethical problems present.

Staff attitudes. Note staff reactions to patient's behaviour. Rapport during interview, interviewer's reactions.

5. Further investigations

Physical investigations as indicated.
Psychological testing.
Psychiatric social worker's report.

6. Formulation of the case

Discuss the differential diagnosis, giving evidence for and against the various possibilities. Make and record a *provisional diagnosis*, an estimate of prognosis, a *problem list*, and plans for *further investigation* and *treatment*.

7. Screening for organic brain disease

This is important in all psychiatric patients and in neurological, geriatric and general medical and surgical patients. The most effective questions are given below. They are simple, do not take long to administer, and give an accurate positive or negative result in nearly all cases. Organic brain disease is usually missed simply by failing to examine for it. Rough scoring is suggested. Note that attention and general information may be affected in depressed patients. Scores on repeated testing will indicate improvement or deterioration.

Orientation

What is the day of the week, the date, the month, the season, the year?   (5)
What is the name of this place? What kind of place is it?   (2)
What is your name?   (1)

Memory
1. Give name and address:
Mrs. Jean Black, 12 West Street, Bathgate.
Ask patient to repeat. Score (1) for each word.   (7)
Repeat until learned, and record number of trials.
2. Test recall after two minutes.   (7)
If results equivocal repeat — with telephone number 337 6924 or with
Babcock sentence:
'One thing a nation must have to become rich and great is a large
secure supply of wood.' Repeat up to eight times if necessary.

Attention and concentration
Serial Sevens: 100 - 7 = 93, 86, 79, 72, 65.
Stop after five numbers   (5)

General information
President U.S.A., Prime Minister, Monarch, name four Scottish
(English) towns, Beethoven, Wordsworth, Rembrandt.   (7)

Language functions
Name a pen/pencil, watch, watchstrap.   (3)
Repeat the words 'No ifs, ands or buts'.   (1)
Carry out a three-stage command: 'Take this paper in your right hand,
fold it in half and put it on the floor'.   (3)
Read and carry out: 'Close your eyes'.   (1)
Write a sentence.   (1)

Parietal function
Show me your left hand.   (1)
Touch your nose with your right hand.   (1)
Name coin placed in hand.   (1)
Make a square with matches.   (1)
Copy a design, e.g. two intersecting rectangles.   (1)

FURTHER READING

De Paulo J R et al 1980 Psychiatric screening on a neurological ward. Psychological
    Medicine 10: 125-132
Hare M 1978 Clinical check list for diagnosis of dementia. British Medical Journal (22
    July): 266-267
Hinton J, Withers E 1971 The usefulness of the clinical tests of the sensorium. British
    Journal of Psychiatry 119: 1-18

4

Psychological tests

Various tests are used in the examination of the psychiatric patient in order to measure aspects of intelligence or of personality. The administration and scoring of these tests requires expertise and in practice patients are referred to specially trained clinical psychologists who undertake testing as one part of their duties. Clinical psychologists also undertake behaviour therapy with certain patients (see Ch. 22).

Intelligence tests

Tests of general intelligence yielding an intelligence quotient (IQ) are used:

1. In the diagnosis of mental handicap
2. To provide background information about the patient for diagnosis and prognosis
3. In the assessment of the patient for rehabilitation and vocational guidance.

For example, an IQ may help to decide whether a patient's difficulty at work is due to a discrepancy between his intelligence and what is expected of him, or is due to emotional difficulties. The patient's test results are appraised in the light of his educational, occupational and social history.

Examples

Wechsler Adult Intelligence Scale. The IQ is derived from the results of 11 sub-tests. Six of these tests are verbal (i.e. question and answer) and five are performance tests (involving manipulation of test material).

Verbal tests
Vocabulary (defining words)
Information (general knowledge)

Comprehension (commonsense)
Arithmetic (14 mental calculations)
Similarities (categorising similarities between pairs of items)
Digit span (remembering increasing sequences of numbers).

Performance tests
Digit symbol (substituting symbols for numbers)
Picture completion (noting missing items in drawings)
Block design (reproducing diagrams using coloured blocks)
Picture arrangement (arranging pictures in logical sequence)
Object assembly (jigsaws).

This scale yields:

1. An overall measure of intellectual capacity

2. Separate measures of intelligence on verbal and performance scales

3. Indication of the patient's particular intellectual abilities or defects

4. An estimate of the degree of intellectual deterioration.

Progressive Matrices. This test measures intellectual ability using the capacity to reason by understanding relationships. The patient is asked to select from a number of alternatives the design which completes a pattern. Sixty such problems of increasing difficulty are presented to the patient. His score on the test when corrected for age yields a percentile rating (i.e. his relative position for intelligence in a random sample of 100 members of the population).

The test is useful as a quick indicator of a patient's level of intelligence. Because it is non-verbal and self-explanatory it can be used in patients with speech or language difficulties.

The Progressive Matrices gives a measure of general intelligence only when it is combined with a score on the Mill-Hill Vocabulary Scale (a standard list of words arranged in order of difficulty, each of which has to be defined).

Measuring intellectual deterioration

In psychiatric illnesses various types of intellectual handicap may occur (see Ch. 6). In dementia the intellectual loss may be assessed clinically by comparing the patient's present performance with the pre-illness level of functioning judged from school and occupational history. A more accurate measurement of intellectual deterioration can be achieved by using the results of the tests which are known to be resistant to intellectual loss, for example vocabulary tests, as indicators of the pre-illness level of intelligence, and noting the discrepancy between these resistant test-scores and the scores on tests which are sensitive to deterioration. For example, comparing the patient's score on Mill-Hill Vocabulary Scale (resistant) with his score on Progressive Matrices (sensitive) gives a measure of the degree of intellectual deterioration over and above that expected for his age.

In addition, special tests are used to elicit specific intellectual changes such as: memory loss (Wechsler Clinical Memory Scale and Benton Visual Retention test), perceptual disturbances (Bender Gestalt test), disturbance of abstract thinking (Goldstein Scherer test), learning difficulties (Paired Associate Learning Test).

The *Halstead-Reitan Neuropsychological Test Battery* consists of a large number of tests of the patient's intellectual, motor and speech functions. It includes tests of thinking, orientation, perception of rhythm and speech, tactile recognition, aphasia as well as general intelligence and takes several hours to administer to a patient. Performance on all the individual tests is combined to give an index of intellectual impairment and analysis of results can give indications of localisation of the central nervous system lesion.

The *Crichton Geriatric Scale* consists of a group of tests designed to discriminate between functional and organic conditions in the elderly. As well as containing a standard IQ test for the elderly, this scale includes an orientation test and a test measuring the patient's ability to detect simultaneous two-point sensory stimulation (the Face-Hand test).

For a clinical screening test for organic conditions, see page 12.

Tests of thinking

Two tests used to measure abnormal thinking in schizophrenic patients are the *Payne Classification Test* and the *Bannister Grid Test for Schizophrenic Thought Disorder*. The former is made up of a number of objects, varying according to size, shape, colour, etc., which the patient is asked to group in any way he likes. There are a number of acceptable (normal) groupings, and any grouping outwith this is termed 'overinclusive', and indicates that the person is using a wide and unusual classificatory system when he thinks.

The *Bannister Repertory Grid Test* measures how well integrated and consistent a person's thinking is. It consists of a number of pictures of male and female faces which the patient is required to order according to the degree to which they possess certain personality traits, e.g. kind, sincere, etc. This test correlates highly with psychiatric ratings of thought disorder in schizophrenic patients, who typically show loose and inconsistent thinking on this test.

Personality tests

Questionnaires

The patient can be asked to complete or tick answers to a list of questions about his attitudes, habits and ways of behaving. For example, the PEN inventory developed by Eysenck produces scores on three dimensions of personality. Psychoticism (ranging from strong contact with reality to impersonal withdrawal), Extraversion (ranging from outgoing sociality to shut-in Introversion), and Neuroticism (ranging from emotional stability to instability). Questionnaires are generally too inaccurate for individual clinical work but may be of value in investigating the personality characteristics of groups of patients. Many others are in use, some measuring diagnostic categories and others personality traits.

The *Minnesota Multiphasic Personality Inventory* (MMPI) is used in psychiatric diagnosis. The patient is asked to judge whether each of 550 statements applies to himself. These statements cover a wide spectrum of mental and somatic complaints, habits, attitudes and moods. The patient's responses are converted into a profile covering 10 basic scales such as Depression, Paranoia, Hysteria, etc. A scoring method is available to detect exaggeration or bias in the responses given by the patient.

The *Sixteen Personality Factor Test* (16 PF) measures 16 common personality traits. Unlike the MMPI scales these are not psychiatric but are psychological characteristics, such as self-sufficiency, submissiveness, imaginativeness, radical-mindedness, etc. These traits are derived statistically from a factor analysis of 185 questions answered on a Yes/No/Uncertain basis. For each individual an overall personality profile is obtained.

While the 16 PF assesses surface traits, the *Edwards Personal Preference Schedule* (EPPS) attempts to assess an individual's psychological needs. This test measures such characteristics as a need for achievement, need for autonomy, need for order, etc. This need profile may be compared with the actual surface trait profile obtained from the 16 PF.

Other questionnaires try to assess a single personality trait with a high degree of accuracy. Examples of these are the *Fould's Hostility* and *Hysteroid Scales.*

Projective tests

The patient is presented with unstructured or meaningless material such as inkblots (Rorschach test) or vague pictures (Thematic Apperception test) and asked to report what he perceives. The patient's responses to this material are considered to be projections of himself from which the examiner can make inferences about personality. While interesting responses may be obtained, their interpretation is difficult and unreliable, and these tests are less widely used than formerly.

Diagnostic measurement

The imprecision of psychiatric diagnoses and the low diagnostic agreement between psychiatrists has led to the development of many *rating scales.* With the use of careful definitions, and training of those using them, high agreement can be reached, and such instruments are much used in research as are *questionnaires* completed by the patients.

General interview schedules include the *Brief Psychiatric Rating Scale* (BPRS) widely used in drug trials and comprising 18 symptoms rated on a 7 point scale of severity. Computer programmes are available to classify patients by their scores.

The *Present State Examination* (PSE) covers a detailed clinical interview in 140 items and gives a score on 38 syndromes. A CATEGO computer programme gives a standardised diagnosis. It is widely used as a research instrument in international studies of schizophrenia.

The *Standard Psychiatric Interview* (SPI) takes less time and is widely used in distinguishing psychiatric from non-psychiatric cases, e.g. in general practice. Many scales are available for specific disorders, e.g. the Hamilton Rating Scale for depression, the Taylor Manifest Anxiety Scale and the Leyton Obsessional Inventory. The Middlesex Hospital Questionnaire (MHQ) for use in psychoneurosis gives a rapid measurement of symptoms and personality traits.

The *General Health Questionnaire* (GHQ) is an example of an instrument to be completed by patients. It has 60 items which the patient scores on a four-point scale. It identifies non-psychotic psychiatric disorder and gives a measure of severity. Widely used as a screening test in general practice and community surveys.

FURTHER READING

Mowbray R M, Rodger T F 1978 Psychology in relation to medicine. Churchill Livingstone, Edinburgh

5

Epidemiology

The study of disorders in groups and communities is of obvious relevance to psychiatric disorders. Epidemiological methods are likely to be useful in elucidating conditions in which environmental factors play a part and in which multiple causes seem likely. Any positive findings are likely to suggest social preventive measures, e.g. better planning for future services, and government and voluntary action to remedy environmental factors or to protect vulnerable groups of individuals.

Early examples of psychiatric epidemiology include Goldberger's work from 1914 in the Southern United States on the causes of pellagra. He demonstrated by epidemiological field-work that the disease was not infectious but was related to a diet low in animal protein. Epidemiological studies on bomber crews in the 1939-45 war showed that high psychiatric breakdown rates were due to inefficient selection procedures rather than excessively long tours of duty. More recently research, using these techniques, has given useful results in alcoholism, suicide and parasuicide and in the planning of psychiatric services.

Prevalence of psychiatric disorder
For over a century contemporary stresses ranging from railway travel to atomic warfare have been blamed for apparent increases in mental illnesses. There is, in fact, little evidence that the true prevalence of psychiatric disorders has changed greatly in the last century. Studies comparing admissions over as long as 100 years in places where reliable records exist show no real change once corrections are made for the ageing population.

There have been increases, but they have been in hospital admission rates, which do not necessarily measure prevalence in the population as a whole. Increased admissions over the years always follow increased provision of hospital beds or new mental health laws. Changes in legislation have made treatment more easily available and have diminished the stigma attached to it. In the last 40 years the development of effective physical treatments has encouraged admissions. More people are now admitted to psychiatric in-patient care; readmissions are much higher, but rates of stay are shorter. Because of the ageing population there have been steady increases in the last 50 years in the admission rates for affective illness and dementia, both disorders whose incidence increases with age.

Hospital admission rates give a rough measure of the more severe psychiatric disorders. Prevalence today can be estimated more accurately from out-patient attendances, the numbers of psychiatric patients seen in general practice and by community surveys; the wider the net the bigger the catch. When attempts are made to measure the milder disorders, problems of defining a case arise and standardised interviews and questionnaires are necessary if the results are to be meaningful.

Once careful study in general practice showed that of all patients seen, 15 per cent had mild, 3 per cent moderate, and 1.4 per cent severe psychiatric disorders. A further 13 per cent were considered to show some emotional disturbance, making a total of one-third of all patients. A hospital census in England showed that on one day 2.86 per 1000 of the population were hospitalised for psychiatric reasons. Of these, 31 per cent were mentally handicapped and 69 per cent mentally ill. It has been estimated that the individual's lifetime expectancy of a psychiatric admission is 1 in 9 for males and 1 in 6 for females.

Other epidemiological findings

Most research now is carried out on specific conditions rather than psychiatric disorder as a whole. The important findings about suicide, alcoholism, schizophrenia and the affective illnesses will be found in the appropriate chapters. The following findings have some general importance.

Sex

Females have higher admission rates than males, consistently enough to be allowed for in planning bed provision. Probably due largely to increased affective illness and longevity in females.

Age

Admission rates increase with age up to the seventies because of the increased risk from affective illness and dementia.

Marital status

Marriage protects against admission, shortens stay, and increases the chances of discharge.

Urban-rural

Rates are higher in town than in country. The larger the city the higher the rates.

Suburban neurosis

It has been suggested that young housewives in badly planned housing estates have a greater risk of developing psychiatric disorder. There is a vulnerable group of women, but its size is no different in housing estates, new towns and older property in the centre of towns.

Migration

Immigrants and emigrants have higher rates.

National and cultural

Primitive communities are not immune although the culture may colour the symptomatology. There are no major variations among Western countries and the U.S.

Social class

Has been studied in detail for many conditions. Mental illness has a social geography. In the decaying centres of big cities schizophrenia is more prevalent, and this and other disorders (but not affective illness) are associated with areas of social disorganisation and mobility. Schizophrenia is six times as common in social class 5 as in social class 1, but the increase is due to downward social mobility. Fathers of schizophrenics in social class 5 come from a wide range of social classes. The increase in social class 5 is thus a consequence of illness rather than its cause.

There have been similar arguments about the accumulation of schizophrenic patients in city centres. One view is that the environment causes the disease, the other that schizophrenics, as a result of their illness, 'drift' to decaying areas (the drift hypothesis). There is much evidence to support the drift hypothesis.

Conclusions

Epidemiological studies of psychiatric disorder demonstrate that social disorganisation and isolation are associated with high risks of breakdown. Those at risk in the community include the elderly, those widowed and divorced, the recently bereaved, the unmarried and those living alone or away from home, especially in large cities.

FURTHER READING

Arthur R G 1971 An introduction to social psychiatry. Penguin, Harmondsworth
Kiev A 1972 Transcultural psychiatry. Penguin, Harmondsworth

6

Organic states and epilepsy

Definition of organic states

Organic mental illnesses are caused by anatomical or physiological disturbance occurring primarily in the brain or central nervous system or resulting from physical illness elsewhere in the body. Acute organic states are sometimes called symptomatic psychoses; chronic states are referred to as dementias. The symptomatology varies with the rate of development of the disease process, the position, duration, extent and severity of the damage to the central nervous system, and the premorbid personality and intelligence of the patient.

'Organic' pathology should be suspected where psychiatric symptoms occur in the presence of the following:

1. No positive emotional factors in aetiology
2. History of trauma, toxic factors, familial degenerative disease, etc.
3. Abnormal neurological signs
4. Age over 45 years.

Certain psychological changes are characteristic, e.g. sudden or progressive deterioration of intellectual powers, especially memory, beyond that expected for age and basic intelligence; loss of sensory or motor function; perceptual changes, e.g. loss of spatial perception; disorientation; sudden or progressive change of personality, especially the following — inappropriate mood, euphoria, apathy, lack of concern for others, shallowness of affect, bizarre behaviour, misinterpretations, 'moral deterioration', irritability, 'catastrophic reactions', 'organic orderliness'.

Examination and investigations

A full history should be obtained from the patient and a friend or relative.

Both psychiatric and neurological examinations should be undertaken. For a suggested screening test see page 12. Special attention should be paid to the following features:

Appearance and general behaviour. Consistent with history? Mannerisms, tics, posture. Tidiness and appropriateness of dress.

Mood. Appropriate to the situation. Emotional lability or fixity. Insight. Disinhibition.

Orientation. Time, date, place, person, age, circumstances of hospitalisation. Can he estimate time-intervals and experience continuity in time? Can he orientate himself readily in new surroundings?

Attention. Distractibility or imperturbability. Can he shift from one topic to another? Is his concentration impaired? Does he perseverate?

Memory. Does memory seem intact? Can he remember events of an hour ago, a day ago? Can he remember more remote events? Nature of amnesia, e.g. for names, faces, and whether it is retrograde or anterograde. Confabulations and fabrications. Does spontaneous recall differ from deliberate recall?

Intelligence. General impression. Range of knowledge and expression. Test reading, writing, comprehension. Are abilities consistent with education and level of intelligence? Agraphia, alexia, acalculia. Can he use numbers as concepts?

Speech. Clarity, modulation, articulation, pronunciation, stammering, dysphasia, range of vocabulary and use of words.

Thinking. Abstract and concrete thinking. Can he control the direction of his thinking? Note content.

Personality. In what way has the personality changed from premorbid personality? Interests, motives, inter-personal relationships, ethical sense.

Tests of intellectual deterioration (see p. 15).

Detailed physical examination of the nervous system, serological tests for syphilis, skull X-rays, EEG, lumbar puncture, perimetry, angiography, isotope and EMI scans, etc., as indicated.

Clinical descriptions

In the symptomatic psychoses the most important symptom is *clouding of consciousness.* This is a state of disturbed awareness which may vary from coma to the mildest degree of confusion. EEG changes are present in proportion to the degree of clouding, with slowing of the dominant frequency in most cases.

Acute organic states

Delirium. Symptomatic psychoses in which consciousness is clouded to the extent that the patient is disorientated for time and place. The attention is fleeting and narrowed — the patient is unable to grasp his present situation and relate it to the past. Thinking is concerned with imaginary experiences and there may be illusional falsifications and dream-like hallucinations — usually visual. Restlessness and hyperkinesis occur; in extreme cases, muttering delirium. Speech disturbance such as pointless repetition, perseveration and dysarthria are found. The mood is one of fear and bewilderment. Sleep rhythm is disturbed. There may be fits.

In each case the individual pattern, especially the thought content, is determined by the premorbid personality. After recovery there is usually amnesia for the events of the illness. Residual delusions may occur and a paranoid attitude may persist for some time.

Subacute organic states

Dysmnesic syndrome. The principal symptom is a difficulty in retaining recent events. There is vague and faulty orientation, and a varying degree of confabulation. Delirium may return at night. This picture may last from a few days to several months, and often follows a delirium.

Subacute delirious state. A symptomatic psychosis in which the degree of clouding is less deep and less constant than in delirium. Incoherence of thought and speech appear, together with perplexity, in a setting of clouding of consciousness which fluctuates in degree and is worse at night. The illness may last for weeks but normally ends in recovery.

Chronic organic states

Dementia. Usually defined as an irreversible decline of mental functions produced by organic brain disease. The process may be arrested; e.g. in neurosyphilis, vitamin deficiencies, some brain tumours. The most obvious finding is intellectual deterioration, but emotion and volition are also impaired. The earliest changes are difficulty in recent memory, failing attention and slow, laboured, vague thinking. At first, symptoms are concealed by memory aids, confabulation, etc. The mood is labile, shallow and blunted, and finally fatuous and euphoric. Judgement, self-control and initiative are all impaired. Sudden unpredictable and disproportionate reaction to frustration (the catastrophic reaction), organic orderliness and denial of illness are found. Psychological testing shows loss of normal perceptual ability (e.g. to distinguish figure and ground) and the presence of concrete thinking.

Atypical organic states

These are conditions which, instead of showing the usual organic symptoms listed above, mimic other mental illnesses, notably mania, depression and schizophrenia. Examples include the psychoses associated with abuse of amphetamine drugs, and the schizophreniform psychoses of epilepsy.

Differential diagnosis

If the examination suggested above has been carefully carried out there is usually little difficulty in distinguishing organic from functional states. Rarely, clouding of consciousness may be seen in acute mania and in acute schizophrenic excitement and give rise to difficulty. The only common source of difficulty is in puerperal psychosis where both symptomatic and functional psychoses may coexist.

Classification

Terms like 'delirium' and 'dementia' are descriptive. The following classification is based on aetiology.

Metabolic and nutritional disorders
1. Carbohydrate: functional and secondary hypoglycaemia
2. Vitamin deficiency:
   a. Aneurine hydrochloride (thiamine): Korsakoff's psychosis, Wernicke's encephalopathy
   b. Nicotinic acid: pellagra
   c. Vitamin B_{12}: pernicious anaemia, 'megaloblastic madness'
3. Porphyrins: porphyria
4. Hormones:
   a. Thyroid: thyrotoxicosis, myxoedema
   b. Adrenal: Addison's disease, Cushing's syndrome
   c. Pituitary: Simmonds's disease
5. Oxygen:
   a. Anaesthesia
   b. Pulmonary disease
   c. Poor carrying power (carbon monoxide poisoning, anaemia).
6. Dialysis dementia: aluminium accumulation in chronic dialysis

Cerebro-vascular disorders
1. Multi-infarct dementia: 'arteriosclerotic dementia'
2. Slow cerebral blood flow: cardiac failure
3. Rarer vascular diseases: polyarteritis nodosa, disseminated lupus, temporal arteritis, thrombo-angiitis obliterans
4. Hypertensive encephalopathy.

Mechanical stresses

1. Space occupying lesions (primary and secondary tumour, abscess, etc.)
2. Trauma, acute and chronic (brain damage, subdural haematoma, post-concussional syndrome, 'punch-drunk syndrome').

Infections

1. Meningitis
2. Encephalitis, and subacute spongiform encephalopathies
3. Syphilis: general paralysis of the insane (G.P.I.)
4. Others, e.g. typhoid, cysticercosis, toxoplasmosis.

Intoxications

1. Exogenous
   a. Medication — e.g. reactions to sedatives, stimulants, chemotherapy, hormones, hypotensive drugs, antihistamines, antidepressants, steroids, digitalis
   b. Self-administered — alcohol, drugs, e.g. barbiturates, cannabis, L.S.D., etc.
   c. Occupational — lead, manganese, methyl chloride, carbon disulphide, etc.
2. Endogenous
   Renal failure; liver failure

Degenerative disorders

1. Senile dementia.
2. Presenile dementia — simple, Huntington's chorea, Alzheimer's, Pick's and Creutzfeld-Jakob's diseases.

Epilepsy

Idiopathic and secondary, especially temporal lobe epilepsy.
Psychomotor attacks.
Post-ictal psychotic episodes (twilight states).
Epileptic dementia and personality change.

Clinical features

Alcohol

Delirium tremens. Usually occurs after intercurrent disease or sudden withdrawal of alcohol in a chronic addict. Clinically there is restlessness, insomnia and an affect of intense fear, with visual hallucinations, illusions and extreme distractibility. Coarse generalised tremor, tachycardia and excessive perspiration are typical.

Treatment is by attention to fluid balance, sedation, vitamins.

Alcoholic dementia. There is gradual intellectual and moral deterioration. The affect is shallow and labile. Although socially pleasant, the patient is often domestically querulous and jealous. The process is arrested but not reversed by abstention.

Korsakoff's psychosis. A dysmnesic syndrome with disorientation, hallucinations, memory loss for recent events and disordered time sense. The patient compensates for his memory loss by describing fictitious events — *confabulation.* There is an associated peripheral neuritis. Associated with lesions of the mammillary bodies and third ventricle.

Infections

General paralysis of the insane. Syphilis: symptoms occur on the average 10 years after the primary infection and the onset is between the ages of 30 and 45. Neurological examination shows dysarthria, tremor of face, lips and tongue, and Argyll-Robertson pupils. Later there may be spastic paralysis and epileptic fits.

Mental symptoms: there is an insidious deterioration of personality with an early loss of finer feelings. The patient becomes irritable, self-centred, less considerate of others and sexually and emotionally disinhibited. Recent memory is impaired. At this stage he may manage to cope with routine tasks but fails if judgement or initiative is required. There is depression or apathy and delusions of grandeur may develop. The disease, if untreated, proceeds to profound dementia and death.

Treatment is by penicillin. Ideally, by prevention: treating the primary infection.

Prognosis is good if diagnosed and treated early enough, although some personality defect will remain.

Fifty years ago one of the most common causes of dementia. Now rare because of treatment of primary infection and so diagnosis may be overlooked. May present with depression or simple dementia.

Encephalitis. In the acute stage there is delirium and there may be convulsions or neurological signs. In post-encephalitic states there is Parkinsonism, apathy and loss of initiative. In children marked personality and intellectual changes may follow the acute stage, resulting in aggressive and antisocial behaviour which may require institutional care. Milder degrees of personality change may also be found. The initial encephalitic illness may not have been severe and diagnosis is often missed. Serial antibody studies may clarify diagnosis.

Degenerative disorders

A formidable social problem created by the ageing population and by the fact that 5 per cent of over 65s develop moderate, and another 5 per cent severe dementia. Presenile dementias (under 65 years) are rare — 0.1 per cent incidence in the general population.

Senile dementia. Loss of neurones is crucial to the clinical symptoms. Other pathological changes consist of *senile plaques* and *neurofibrillary tangles*; the so-called Alzheimer changes first described in Alzheimer's disease. The symptoms are an exaggeration of the normal psychological changes of old age. The patient becomes narrow and restricted in outlook. Memory impairment is an early sign. There is increasing difficulty in comprehension. There is confusion and disorientation, especially at night. Later there is blunting of emotion and apathy. The condition is progressive and death usually occurs in a few years.

Multi-infarct dementia. Dementia associated with vascular disease. Formerly attributed to cerebral arteriosclerosis but correlation with pathology not high, and the multiple infarcts found may be due to thrombotic episodes arising from the heart and large vessels. Occurs at younger ages than senile dementia and is associated with male sex and hypertension.

Memory loss is patchy, less general than in senile dementia, and until the later stages personality and insight are well preserved. The rate of deterioration varies and is erratic — 'step-ladder' progression. Emotional lability common. May be associated with focal signs — hemiparesis, dysphasia, pseudo-bulbar palsy. Depressive and paranoid symptoms common, particularly in early stages, and may initially respond to treatment.

Parkinsonism. His original 1817 description of shaking palsy did *not* include dementia as a symptom, but in a third of cases — especially arteriosclerotic — there is intellectual deterioration. The term *subcortical dementia* has been proposed for these and similar cases where the intellectual changes are associated with akinesia and motor slowing.

Presenile dementias. Alzheimer's disease: A presenile disease with the neuropathology described for senile dementia. The commonest presenile dementia, twice as common in women. Death in 2 to 3 years. Diffuse atrophy especially affecting frontal and temporal cortex.

Early memory defect. Later blunting and irritability. Later epilepsy, parietal lobe signs (agnosia, apraxia).

Pick's disease: Rare. Twice as many women. Early personality change: fatuous, loss of social restraint, apathy. Early loss of insight, dysphasia, incontinence. Later memory loss and intellectual deterioration. Patchy atrophy, especially frontal and temporal lobes. Histopathology — specific changes now disputed.

Huntington's chorea: Rare presenile dementia with choreiform movements. Personality changes precede dementia. Unsteadiness and clumsiness often disguised as clowning. Atrophy of frontal lobe and caudate nucleus.

Inherited as autosomal dominant with full penetrance. Associated with reduced glutamic-acid-decarboxylase activity.

Creutzfeld-Jakob disease: An extremely rare presenile dementia first described in Germany, 1920, with symptoms of cortico-stria-spinal degeneration, myoclonus and a characteristic EEG and death in one year. It is a *subacute spongiform viral encephalopathy* like *scrapie* (a disease of sheep), transmissible mink encephalopathy and *kuru*. The latter is a neurological disease, now dying out, affecting the Fore tribe in highland New Guinea, thought to have been transmitted by cannibalistic eating of the dead. The neuropathology of these conditions shows swellings of neurons and glia, with displacement of the nucleus to the side of the cell. This status spongiosus is intra-cellular.

Creutzfeld-Jakob disease has been transmitted accidentally in humans by a corneal graft and by implanted brain electrodes, and experimentally to chimpanzees and cats. Brain research workers and patients undergoing brain and opthalmic surgery are not at risk if sensible precautions are taken.

Normal pressure hydrocephalus (Adam's syndrome): Rare treatable condition. Non-specific dementia with ataxia and incontinence. Enlarged ventricles and no cerebral atrophy. Previous history of head injury, meningitis or subarachnoid haemorrhage leading to adhesions and obstruction to flow of CSF. CSF shunt operation may lead to improvement.

Trauma

Head injury. A costly epidemic arising from road traffic accidents. Heavy drinkers over-represented. About 100 000 annually in U.K. of whom 1000 become severely disabled. Although physical and social sequelae may be severe, psychological changes are the most disabling. Duration of post-traumatic amnesia is an early guide to severity.

A variety of syndromes because of the many determining factors:
1. Premorbid personality, intelligence, alcohol consumption
2. Amount and location of brain damage
3. Emotional impact of injury
4. Compensation/litigation

5. Post-traumatic epilepsy
6. Environmental factors (occupation, family support)

Minor head injury. The *post-concussional* syndrome is common, especially in injuries where compensation is involved. Symptoms include headache, dizziness, fatigue, sensitivity to noise and small amounts of alcohol, irritability, insomnia, poor concentration and memory. Aetiology disputed: may be both organic and psychological factors in aetiology. Can be very disabling. Usually improves when compensation claim settled. Not associated with severe head injury.

Severe head injuries. The disability includes a mixture of:

a. generalised intellectual impairment, with slowing, apathy, poor memory and concentration. May be catastrophic reaction. Slow improvement may take place up to 20 years after injury.

b. focal abnormalities e.g. language difficulties, Korsakoff syndrome, agnosias, apraxias, etc.

c. Personality change, especially frontal lobe syndrome (facile euphoria, tactlessness, disinhibition), explosive aggressive personality, and depression or anxiety with temporal lobe injury.

d. Psychoses — rarely.

Punch drunkenness. A syndrome of dementia with minor neurological signs in boxers who have fought too many unsuccessful fights. Associated with abnormalities of the septum pellucidum. Rarer than those opposed to the sport suggest.

Space occupying lesions

Includes tumours (primary and secondary), subdural haematoma, cysts, etc. The usual symptoms are apathy, blunting of feeling and a reduction of alertness. There may be memory difficulty and impulsive behaviour. These symptoms are caused by the rise of intracranial pressure and have no localising value. Focal neurological signs may or may not be present. In some cases affective or schizophrenic illness may be mimicked.

Miscellaneous

In *myxoedema* there is apathy, retardation of thinking, poor memory and reduced intellectual ability. In addition the patient may be depressed or paranoid. *Thyrotoxicosis* may produce a mixture of anxiety, affective and organic symptoms. Mental symptoms may also occur in deficiency diseases, e.g. *pellagra*, and in chronic systematic diseases, e.g. evening delirium in *congestive heart failure,* intellectual deterioration and euphoria in *multiple sclerosis.* Acute confusional symptoms or an 'hysterical' syndrome may occur in *porphyria.* In elderly patients minor degrees of physical illness (e.g. anaemia, chest or bladder infection, cardiac failure) may precipitate a confusional state. Toxic manifestations are also commonly associated with the use of sedatives and stimulant drugs. Barbiturates and amphetamines are particularly liable to cause confusion.

Confusion, excitement and sometimes hallucinations may be either idiosyncratic reactions or follow excessive dosage as in addiction. Some cases of amphetamine psychosis closely resemble acute paranoid schizophrenia.

Epilepsy

Epilepsy is the spontaneous paroxysmal discharge of excitation in the central nervous system. The resulting symptoms range from major convulsions with complete loss of consciousness to momentary tics with brief lapse of consciousness. Causal factors include neoplastic, hereditary, traumatic, infective and circulatory. Epilepsy is therefore not a disease entity but a symptom requiring investigation.

Incidence is difficult to assess because of the difficulty of establishing criteria, controlling age-factors, and of obtaining large-scale figures. A figure of 1/200 is generally accepted.

There are two main forms:

1. *Primary* or *idiopathic*, where the disturbance originates in the centrencephalic system
2. *Secondary* or *focal*, where the disturbance originates from a cortical focus and spreads to the centrencephalic system.

Clinical forms

Grand mal: 'major epilepsy' with definite loss of consciousness. The sequence is generally prodrome (e.g. irritability, restlessness), aura, convulsion, total loss of consciousness (with tonic spasm, followed by clonic jerkings). Disorientation, automatisms, explosive irritability, fugues, furor and twilight states may follow the fit.

Petit mal: 'minor epilepsy' with a characteristic 'absence' or transient loss of consciousness. Akinetic and myoclonic seizures may also occur. The patient is often unaware of the attack. Usually begins in childhood.

Psychical seizures. Forced thinking, déjà vu, hallucinations, illusions and perceptual anomalies are found in these attacks and are usually due to disturbance in the *temporal lobe*, as are:

Psychomotor attacks: partial loss of consciousness, semi-purposive movements. Masticatory movements are common. Twilight states with altered consciousness can be regarded as prolonged psychomotor attacks. Fugues may occur.

Reflex epilepsy: fits precipitated by sensory stimulation, e.g. music, bright colours, touch or flickering light (television).

Epileptic equivalents: emotional instability, compulsive actions, paroxysmal pains, 'thalamic' laughter, behaviour disorders are in rare cases akin to epileptic disorders.

Investigations
  1. *History*
  2. *Physical examination of the nervous system*
  3. *Electroencephalography.* The EEG has contributed greatly to the study of epilepsy. Characteristic generalised spike and wave potentials, or focal spike potentials, may be noted. High amplitude dysrhythmic patterns of very fast and very slow activity may also be seen.

The EEG is a useful aid in investigating epilepsy, in indicating the existence of a focus and in assessing the need for further investigation and treatment. A normal record does not exclude epilepsy and the diagnosis ultimately rests on the history and observation of the seizure.

Treatment
  1. Anticonvulsant medication. Most anticonvulsants can now be monitored in the serum. If adequate levels of one drug are achieved multiple drug therapy is rarely necessary. Phenytoin, phenobarbitone and primidone are used for major seizures. Carbamazepine is useful for focal fits, ethosuximide and sodium valproate for petit mal attacks with typical 3 Hz spike-and-wave EEG abnormalities.
  2. Advice on occupation and recreation, e.g. avoiding alcohol and risks such as driving or working near moving machinery.
  3. Neurosurgery in certain cases of focal epilepsy.

Psychiatric aspects of epilepsy

Associated behaviour disorders and psychoses
In temporal lobe epilepsy, in addition to major seizures (in 50 per cent of cases), psychic and psychomotor attacks, there can be *behaviour disturbance* between the attacks. This is usually in the form of aggressive hostile behaviour, but paranoid, depressive and hysterical symptoms occur. In these cases the so-called *epileptic personality* may be seen. Such patients are self-centred, morose and religiose, and are pedantic and laborious both in speech and thought. *Psychoses* closely mimicking schizophrenia are seen in some cases. Temporal lobe epilepsy accounts for about one-third of all cases of epilepsy.

Epileptic dementia

In severe and uncontrolled epilepsy intellectual deterioration can occur over the years and lead to dementia. This must be distinguished from the temporary and reversible effects of seizures on memory (cf. ECT) and from the cumulative effects of large doses of anticonvulsants, especially phenobarbitone.

Psychological reactions to epilepsy

Although only a few show mental disturbances most epileptics have psychological problems due to their illness and to society's attitude to the disorder, which is still regarded with superstition and fear. As it is not in their best interests to work machines or drive, epileptic patients have difficulties in finding employment and may become discouraged. Encouragement, help and interest are essential.

FURTHER READING

Corsellis J A N et al 1973 The aftermath of boxing. Psychological Medicine 3: 270-303

Lishman W A 1973 The psychiatric sequelae of head injury: a review. Psychological Medicine 3: 304-318

Lishman W A 1978 Organic psychiatry. Blackwell, Oxford

7

Affective disorders

The term affective disorder covers illnesses in which disturbance of affect (mood) is the primary symptom; all other symptoms are secondary. The mood may be persistently depressed or elated (in mania) and episodes of either type may occur in the same person, hence the term 'manic-depressive psychosis'. Illnesses with only one type of attack are called unipolar; with both manic and depressive episodes, bipolar. All these are primary depressions. Secondary depressions may follow other psychiatric disorders or physical illness (see Table 1).

Table 1 Classification of depressive illness

1. Primary

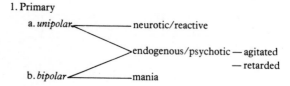

2. Secondary

    a. to physical illness

    b. to psychiatric illness

Aetiology

Genetics. Twin studies show concordance rates of 70 per cent for monozygotic twins and 20 per cent for dizygotic twins. The incidence in the general population is 1 per cent and in first degree relatives 10-15 per cent. The type of transmission is probably polygenic, leading to varying degrees of predisposition. Bipolar and unipolar illnesses breed true.

Biochemistry. Inherited disorders must have biochemical origins. Various changes have been found in depressed patients, including increased adrenocortical activity and altered distribution of water and electrolytes, but the *monoamine theory* has provoked most research.

There are three brain mono-amines — dopamine, noradrenaline and serotonin (5-hydroxytryptamine or 5 HT). The drug reserpine depletes the brain of mono-amines and may cause depression. There is evidence of altered 5 HT metabolism in depression. Some antidepressant drugs are mono-amine oxidase inhibitors (MAOI), and may work by increasing the concentration of mono-amines in the brain. The theory proposes that depression may be due to a decreased concentration of mono-amines at receptor sites in the brain.

Sex incidence. Affective illness is twice as common in women and is frequently associated with the puerperium and the menopause. Suicide and admission to hospital are more frequent premenstrually. During affective illness amenorrhoea often occurs. These factors suggest that an endocrine disturbance may be of aetiological importance.

Premorbid personality. Mild disturbances of mood are usual. Cyclothymic personalities are subject to mild swings of mood throughout life, unrelated to external causes. Depressive personalities are habitually gloomy, pessimistic and lacking in drive. Hypomanic personalities are habitually more cheerful, energetic and sociable than average.

Body build. Affective illness is often associated with the *pyknic body build*, stocky, round-faced, with thick short neck, fat trunk and slender extremities — the John Bull physique.

Age. The incidence rises with increasing age.

Seasonal influence. There is a higher incidence of affective illness and suicide in the late spring and early summer.

Social class. Affective illness is more frequent in the higher social classes.

Infection and drugs. Depressive illness often follows virus infections, particularly influenza and hepatitis, and may follow the administration of reserpine, methyldopa and steroids and oral contraceptives.

Childhood. Depressed patients have more often lost a parent in childhood than the rest of the population.

Loss. The usual precipitant of affective illness is the loss of a loved object. This may range from the serious (loss of spouse, employment, status, health, or self-respect) to the apparently trivial — loss of a pet.

Depression

Clinical picture

Psychological symptoms. There is a general loss of vitality which the patient may express as a loss of interest, or lack of energy. The patient appears tired and sad. Usually he withdraws from social activities and from people and his activity declines at work and in the home. The degree of depression can be slight or profound. Everything seems gloomy and hopeless. Anxiety may be present or the patient may try to conceal his symptoms ('smiling depression').

Diurnal variation. All symptoms tend to be worse in the early morning and improve as the day goes on.

Suicide. May be first sign of the illness. The risk of suicide is difficult to assess but is always present. Suicidal ideas should always be enquired about and taken seriously when elicited. Rarely, depressives may kill their relatives believing they must save them from a life of misery.

Retardation or slowing of thinking is usual, and is reflected in speech and movement. There is poverty of thought and difficulty in concentration. Rarely retardation can be severe enough to produce stupor. *Agitation* may be the dominant symptom in other cases, with obvious motor restlessness, pacing the floor and wringing of hands. There is accompanying anxiety, speech is increased in amount but the content is repetitious, and poverty of thought remains.

Feelings of guilt are usual, with self-reproach and self-depreciation. In severe cases delusions may develop; the illness is regarded as a punishment for past sins, real or imagined. The patient may feel that he is despised and accused of sinfulness by others. There is self-absorption, hypochondriasis and hypochondriacal delusions may occur. There may also be delusions of poverty or nihilistic delusions.

Hallucinations are rare but can occur in severe cases.

Depersonalisation and derealisation are not infrequent. The patient states that he has lost his feelings and has sensations of strangeness. He feels unreal and things look unreal to him. *Obsessional* thoughts and actions, usually with a content of guilt or self-blame, may be found.

Physical symptoms

Insomnia is usual. Typically the patient wakens early, but later both early and late insomnia and even total insomnia follow.

Anorexia, constipation, indigestion, weight loss, amenorrhoea and *loss of libido* are usual. Any of these may be the original presenting symptom. Hypochondriacal concern with such symptoms is common. Some depressions may present with unusual single symptoms, such as facial pain.

Summary

The typical symptoms of depression are loss of vitality, sadness, retardation, poverty of thought, self-depreciation, hopelessness, self-absorption, late insomnia and diurnal variation.

Types of depression

The symptoms described above are those of *endogenous* depression, i.e. depression arising from internal causes, genetic and biochemical. They respond to physical methods of treatment, and may run a bipolar course. *Neurotic (reactive) depressions* are twice as common but less clear-cut in their symptoms. They are usually less severe, related in time to a significant loss, and respond temporarily to reassurance, a change of environment or company. The typical sleep disturbance and diurnal variation of endogenous depression is rare and associated neurotic symptoms are common. They can be seen to stem from neurotic personality problems worsened or reactivated by obvious precipitants. They respond less well to physical treatment, and require psychotherapy (see p. 82).

The classification of depression has provoked much argument and research. One school of thought considers that the two types described are entirely different in quality, the other that the two patterns are at the extremes of a normal distribution curve with most patients falling between them. Whatever the truth, the two types described are valuable in predicting response to treatment.

Mania

Clinical picture

Mania is rarer than depression. The patient feels perfectly well physically and mentally and is usually brought to the doctor by his family. The mood is euphoric, with flashes of irritability, and varies from mild elation to wild hilarity and excitement. The patient's cheerfulness is infectious but quickly becomes tiresome. There is increased mental and physical activity; less sleep is required and there is talkativeness and over-optimistic planning for the future. The patient is tactless and disinhibited, and may be promiscuous and extravagant.

Thinking. The stream of thought is rapid but rarely to the point. Thinking is not directed logically but by casual association, e.g. sounds, puns, rhymes (flight of ideas).

Attention cannot be sustained for any time.

Delusions when present are usually grandiose and unsustained. Severe cases may be *disorientated* and *restless* so that physical exhaustion may be a risk to life.

Course and prognosis

Affective disorders are common. In a 10 year period in general practice about 1 in every 10 of the practice population will complain of depression. About ten cases of depression are seen for each one of mania.

The typical attack lasts from 6 to 9 months but may range from hours to many years. Complete recovery from the attack is the rule but some 10 per cent become chronic, with permanent or fluctuating mood changes. In depression two-thirds of patients have a single attack, in mania one-half never have a recurrence. In patients who have recurrent attacks most will have repeated attacks of depression, about one in three will be bipolar (both manic and depressive) and only 4 per cent will have repeated attacks of mania. The intervals are irregular and unpredictable, but with increasing number of attacks the time interval tends to diminish.

Favourable prognostic features and indicators of good response to physical treatment include typical endogenous symptoms, an abrupt onset, a stable premorbid personality without neurotic traits, and paradoxically, severity of the attack. Unfavourable features include depersonalisation, hypochondriasis, hysterical traits and atypical symptoms of any kind.

Differential diagnosis
Complaints of depression are made in many illnesses. Organic states, especially cerebral tumour and arteriosclerosis, may present with depressive symptoms. In adolescents or young adults depression may be an early symptom of schizophrenia.

The diagnosis of depression may be missed, thereby increasing the risk of suicide. In early cases of depression with predominant anxiety a neurotic illness may be diagnosed. When the presenting symptoms of depression are physical (anorexia, weight loss, loss of libido, etc.) extensive physical investigations may be made and the correct diagnosis delayed.

Hypomania must be differentiated from the effects of stimulant drugs, alcohol, catatonic excitement and the euphoric picture associated with frontal lobe lesions.

Treatment
Electro-convulsive therapy produces remission in over 80 per cent of severe depressions. Antidepressant drugs benefit over 60 per cent of cases but side effects can be troublesome and the delay in response for 2 to 4 weeks is worrying in potentially suicidal patients. ECT and antidepressant drugs are often used in combination. Phenothiazines are used in large doses to control manic symptoms.

These treatments do not prevent further attacks. Long term maintenance treatment with lithium preparations diminishes the frequency and severity of both manic and depressive episodes.

See chapters on treatment.

8

Schizophrenia

Schizophrenia is the most severe form of functional psychosis producing the greatest disorganisation of personality. In severe cases the patient is out of contact with reality to such an extent that his ideas and behaviour are patently abnormal. The illness typically runs a gradual course towards chronicity but may occur in attacks. Complete spontaneous recovery is rare and the untreated disease usually 'burns out' after some years leaving a dilapidated personality — the 'defect state'. The condition was first delineated in 1896 on the basis of its symptoms and natural history by Kraepelin, who used the label dementia praecox. In 1911 Bleuler coined the name schizophrenia to mark the 'splitting' or disruption of psychic function which characterises the illness. There are international differences in diagnostic criteria, especially between Europe and the U.S.A., and many psychiatrists now speak of the 'schizophrenias' as a group of related disorders.

Statistics
The estimated risk of schizophrenia at some time in life is 0.5-1 per cent. Schizophrenia accounts for some 15 per cent of admissions to psychiatric hospitals, for 45 per cent of the hospital population, and the majority of long-stay patients. The disease is more common in males than females and most cases begin before the age of 30.

Symptomatology
A wide range of symptoms occurs in various combinations and at different stages in the course of the disorder. Some are found in other conditions, some are almost confined to schizophrenia and are of greater diagnostic significance.

Disorder of thought
This refers to the form rather than the content: formal thought disorder. Thinking is woolly and diffuse. The normal associations between ideas are disrupted ('knight's move' thinking). The patient

may experience sudden halts in his thinking (thought blocking). Concrete thinking (inability to think in abstract terms) may be demonstrated by asking the patient to give the general meaning of well-known proverbs. Reasoning is disturbed by the intrusion of personal themes (autistic or dereistic thinking), and by inability to select ideas (overinclusive thinking).

Disorder of emotion

The emotional reaction and mood are inappropriate, or incongruous with the patient's situation or thoughts. Later blunting and apathy develop. An early sign is a lack of rapport found at interview.

Disorder of volition

There is a loss of will-power, lassitude and lack of drive, often shown by a falling-off in housework, studying and work. At times excessive obstinacy, negativism or automatic obedience may be found.

Catatonia

Abnormality of movement may occur with awkward, poorly co-ordinated movements and gait, grimacing, posturing and, in extreme cases, waxy flexibility and echopraxia.

Hallucinations

These occur in many illnesses but in schizophrenia are found in a setting of clear consciousness. They are usually auditory, but other sensory modalities may be involved.

Delusions

Primary delusions: the sudden appearance of a fully developed delusion from a normal perception which the patient instantly accepts as overwhelmingly convincing.

Secondary delusions are false beliefs arising from other symptoms, e.g. the patient may 'explain' thought disorder by coming to believe that thoughts are being put into his head by an outside agency, or that his thoughts are being interfered with.

Disturbances of expression

Thought disorder and hallucinations are often reflected in speech (neologisms, word salad), mannered handwriting, and unusual paintings and poems.

Withdrawal

As a result of the above symptoms, withdrawal from normal social contacts and activities is often an early symptom.

Diagnosis

Negative findings are important. Manic or depressive symptoms, or a previous history of them, should be absent. There should be no history of alcohol or drug abuse which might account for the symptoms. Consciousness must be clear, memory and orientation intact. If delusions or hallucinations are not present, convincing thought disorder must be demonstrated. Epilepsy must be excluded.

Schizophrenia can then be diagnosed with confidence if several of Schneider's *first rank symptoms* can be elicited. These comprise the experiences of thought insertion, thought withdrawal and thought broadcasting; feelings of passivity (i.e. the experience of sensations, emotions or even movements being caused or controlled by an outside agency); voices heard talking about the patient in the third person, voices giving a running commentary on the patient's thoughts or behaviour, voices heard to be voicing the patient's own thoughts; and lastly, primary delusions.

In many early cases the diagnosis is doubtful. The premorbid personality and family history may give supporting evidence, but often the progress of the condition must be observed for some time to clarify the diagnosis.

The difficulty of firm diagnosis in the early stages has led many research workers to use structured interviews and computer analysis. Wing's Present State Examination (PSE) with the CATEGO programme has shown that Russian and United States' psychiatrists use a wider definition of the disorder than British psychiatrists. *Operational definitions* are also popular but too rigid for clinical work. As an example Feighner's criteria are:

1. Both required:
   a. Chronic illness of 6 months of symptoms
   b. Absence of affective illness
2. At least one of:
   a. Delusions or hallucinations without perplexity or disorientation
   b. Thought disorder
3. Two for 'probable', three for 'definite' of:
   a. Single
   b. Poor premorbid personality or work record
   c. Positive family history
   d. No alcoholism or drug abuse in last year
   e. Onset before 40.

Clinical picture

The following subtypes of schizophrenia are not separate clinical entities but are convenient methods of classifying schizophrenic reactions.

Hebephrenic schizophrenia. The onset is usually in the late teens. Early symptoms are perplexity, poor concentration, vagueness, daydreaming, self-consciousness, moodiness, depression, apathy, transient delusions, indiscriminate concern with pseudo-scientific and pseudo-philosophical ideas, feelings of inferiority and inadequacy. Thought disturbance becomes obvious and there may be concrete thinking or thought blocking. Emotional incongruity is characteristic.

Paranoid schizophrenia. The typical symptoms are primary and secondary delusions of persecution with auditory hallucinations. The onset is later than in hebephrenic schizophrenia, usually between 30 and 50 years. The course is chronic with minimal deterioration of personality. Misinterpretations of the actions of others may be incorporated in ideas of persecution. The delusions may be 'encapsulated' and the patient may behave normally, but usually his delusional ideas bring him into conflict with society. Although the illness takes a chronic course, there may be periodic fluctuation in the symptoms. The florid illness is often preceded by paranoid traits of personality — hypersensitive or self-conscious individuals who take offence at harmless remarks or who are isolated by reason of deformity, deafness, language difficulty, etc. Sometimes delusional ideas may be 'infectious'; usually a near relative is involved in this *folie à deux.*

Catatonic schizophrenia. Stereotyped behaviour, negativism, posturing, immobility and stupor are the most obvious characteristics. Thought blocking, neologisms, hallucinations may also occur. Acute excitement may be the first sign of the disease. Catatonic symptoms have become increasingly rare in the last 30 years: many may have been a product of institutional neurosis (see p. 109).

Simple schizophrenia. As there are no florid features the diagnosis may be missed for many years. The onset, usually during adolescence, is insidious and the course very slowly progressive. Many cases never reach hospital. Primary symptoms of emotional blunting, loss of volition and thought disorder are usual. The patients drift through life and are solitary; their social level sinks and they may drift into poverty, petty crime, prostitution and vagrancy.

Defect state: the typical picture of chronic schizophrenia shown by many patients both in the community and in long term care. Negative symptoms predominate with lack of drive and initiative, poverty of thought and emotion and solitary, eccentric behaviour. Many show 'age disorientation', and evidence of cerebral damage is accumulating, as shown by dilated cerebral ventricles related in degree to impaired intellectual function.

Aetiology

The cause of schizophrenia is unknown and represents one of the greatest research challenges of contemporary medicine. Much research has already been done and many predisposing and precipitating factors are known.

Heredity. The importance of genetic factors has been convincingly demonstrated. The risk in the general population is 1 per cent, in parents of schizophrenics 5 per cent, in siblings 8 per cent and in children 10 per cent. This last figure persists even when the children have been separated from the parent from birth. The concordance in monozygotic twins is 30-40 per cent.

Environment. These twin figures suggest that environmental factors must play some part in the appearance of the disease in predisposed individuals. Some workers (Laing, Goffman) suggest that schizophrenia is not a disease but a response to intolerable emotional pressures in the family and society, but such extreme views, although fashionable with the public, lack experimental support. Much careful work on childhood influences, particularly on the personalities of the parents, is inconclusive. It has been shown that stresses such as promotion or bereavement are more common in the month preceding the onset or relapses.

Premorbid personality. The previous personality of the patient is often 'schizoid'. This solitary and withdrawn behaviour may explain the large number of single schizophrenics.

Physique. Many schizophrenics are of asthenic build and in the established case there may be poor peripheral circulation, cold cyanotic extremities, and amenorrhoea.

Biochemistry. LSD psychosis and amphetamine psychosis both have some resemblance to schizophrenia; various drugs, particularly phenothiazines, are effective in treating schizophrenia. These 'clues' have led to much research and several theories. Serotin deficiency was the first — LSD blocks serotonin receptors. Dopamine overactivity has been suggested because amphetamines increase dopamine release and drugs for schizophrenia block dopamine receptors. Increased sensitivity of the post-synaptic receptors is the likeliest explanation. Other theories include noradrenaline neurone degeneration, and monoamine oxidase deficiency. No conclusive evidence has emerged. Numerous minor defects of metabolism have been found. In periodic catatonia, a rare condition, nitrogen retention occurs.

Immunology. There is current interest in the role of brain antibodies in the genesis of schizophrenia.

Brain damage. Recent evidence of dilated cerebral ventricles and age disorientation in chronic schizophrenia make an organic cause likely.

Course and prognosis

Schizophrenia is not fatal except through suicide. The general trend is towards disintegration of the personality, but the process may be arrested at any point, leaving a personality defect which may be inconspicuous or obvious. The remission rate without treatment was about 20 per cent, but with treatment some two-thirds make a social recovery. In the past two-thirds of schizophrenics spent their lives in hospital, today fewer than one in ten require permanent hospital care.

Favourable prognostic factors include absence of family history of the disease, normal personality, and stable family background and work record. Features of the illness associated with a good outcome include acute onset, obvious precipitants, retention of normal emotional response, presence of catatonic symptoms, retention of drive and initiative. Early treatment assists a favourable outcome.

Relapse is often associated with increased 'life events' in the preceding three weeks, and occurs more often when the patient is subject to hostility and criticism from relatives. Those on maintenance drugs are three times less likely to relapse than controls, but even with maintenance phenothiazines up to 50 per cent relapse within two years.

Differential diagnosis

Schizophrenia must be distinguished from:

1. Psychological difficulties of *normal adolescence*. This may be especially difficult in shy, sensitive and highly intelligent students.

2. *Symptomatic schizophrenia*. In several conditions, notably psychoses associated with temporal-lobe epilepsy and amphetamine addiction, the symptoms may be indistinguishable from those of schizophrenia.

3. *Affective psychoses*. Some atypical depressions or manias may give rise to diagnostic difficulty. When doubt exists and affective symptoms are prominent the term *schizo-affective psychosis* is sometimes used.

4. Paranoid psychosis produced by *alcoholism*, or the early symptoms of an *organic dementia* may mimic schizophrenia.

Treatment

In the acute phase phenothiazine drugs are given in large doses, often with ECT. Phenothiazines are effective in reducing delusions, hallucinations and disturbed thinking and behaviour, but less effective in altering negative symptoms such as emotional blunting and loss of volition. Maintenance therapy must be given over years and relapse rates are high when attempts are made to stop drugs. As many patients fail to take oral medication regularly, long acting preparations (e.g. fluphenazine decanoate) given every two to four weeks are widely used.

Social therapy is necessary. Schizophrenics require intensive rehabilitation, social and industrial, but the amount of stimulation must be matched to individual requirements. Excessive stimulation has been shown to lead to relapse, too little to continuing withdrawal and chronicity. Rehabilitation must be planned, sometimes over several years, and involves the services of nurses, social workers, occupational therapists and recreational therapists. A variety of facilities is also necessary, ranging from night wards, day hospitals and industrial therapy units to lengthy courses of training in rehabilitation units, and hostel accommodation in the community.

FURTHER READING

Creer C, Wing J 1975 Living with a schizophrenic patient. British Journal of Hospital Medicine 14: 73-82

Kendell R E 1972 Schizophrenia: the remedy for diagnostic confusion. British Journal of Hospital Medicine 8: 383-390

Laing R D 1960 The divided self. Penguin, Harmondsworth

9

Personality disorder and psychopathy

Personality development
Significant temperamental differences found between infants in the
first weeks of life persist at three years of age. This suggests that some
components of personality are genetically determined. Just as
monozygotic twins are closer to each other on intelligence tests scores
than are dizygotic twins, so higher correlations are found between
identical twins on measures of introversion – extraversion and
anxiety.

Such basic differences have further consequences. The sociable
baby and child will be treated differently from the shy, the anxious
differently from the calm, leading to even more pronounced
personality differences. At all stages of early development personality
deviations can be created, e.g. by perinatal damage, by lack of bonding
in early childhood, and by life events such as bereavement in later
childhood.

Normal personality
In adult life there is no single, accepted method of measuring
personality or of classifying types of personality. It is widely agreed
that various dimensions of personality can be identified and measured,
and that the two main dimensions are anxiety level (neuroticism) and
extraversion – introversion (sociability). It has been traditional
among psychiatrists to label types of personality originally observed in
the premorbid personality associated with certain psychiatric
disorders.

Personality disorder
Many individuals whose personalities deviate from the average come
to the attention of doctors and social agencies or into conflict with
society and the law. Those who suffer by being unusual personalities
or who make others suffer are usually said to have personality
disorders. Note that such abnormalities of personality are on a
continuum and are statistical deviations from the average. Just as there

is a continuum of intelligence, so there is a continuun of irritability, sociability, orderliness, etc. Extreme deviations, like genius in relation to intelligence, do not imply illness.

So many labels are attached to personality disorders by psychiatrists, and agreement about their classification is so low, that many believe labelling is unhelpful and should be replaced by a multi-dimensional description of each individual, e.g. scores for neuroticism, extraversion, obsessionality and so on.

The term 'moral insanity' was first used by Pritchard in 1835 to describe 'persons of a singular, wayward and eccentric character'. Other terms which have been used include neurotic character, character disorder, sociopathy, and psychopathic personality. The International Statistical Classification of Diseases favours *personality disorder* with various sub-divisions. These include the types described below.

Problems of 'sociopathy'
There are dangers in regarding these labels as diagnoses. Many deviations of personality are assets and only become defects when carried to extremes, e.g. tidiness. There are particular problems in relation to *responsibility*; deviant personalities are usually responsible for their actions although most psychiatrists would argue that true psychopathic personalities have diminished responsibility in law. There is a great danger that a society, particularly an authoritarian one, will label as deviant or 'sociopathic' any who disagree with its policies, and use the label as an excuse to deprive individuals of their liberty.

Varieties of personality disorder

Cyclothymic (affective)
These individuals show persistent deviations of mood insufficient to be labelled illness. They may be persistently cheerful, talkative, energetic and the life and soul of the party — *hypomanic personalities*; or persistently gloomy, pessimistic, lacking in energy and over-concerned about their health — *depressive personalities*. A third type has frequent or excessive swings of mood, in both directions, lasting long or short periods: true *cyclothymia*. All three types are prone to develop affective illness (q v).

Schizoid
This type of personality, a common precursor of schizophrenia and often seen in the relatives of schizophrenics, is introverted and withdrawn. Because of their aloof and reserved manner they have few friends and are solitary rather than shy. Often intelligent, their lack of

feeling prevents them making close relationships (Belloc's 'remote and ineffectual' dons). They may behave eccentrically in public because of their lack of interest in others.

Paranoid

Personalities, often with schizoid features, who make excessive use of projection as a defence mechanism. They blame others excessively, feeling sensitive and downtrodden and attributing their failure in life to others. Often aggressive, suspicious and irritable individuals, ever ready to take offence and sometimes resorting to litigation in defence of over-valued ideas (querulous litigants).

Hysterical

Hysterical personalities are dramatic, scene-loving, and attention-craving, emotionally shallow and insincere, sexually titillating, but basically frigid. They tend to manipulate their families and friends and can be recognised by their provocative manner and dress, and by their dramatic gestures and extravagant use of language. The personality seems to lack a central core and appears as a series of changing, dramatic masks. More common in women, often working on the stage or otherwise in the public eye.

Obsessional

Long recognised clinically and confirmed by questionnaire and rating scale studies. Two main factors: one of persistence, orderliness and thoroughness; and another of indecision, doubt and uncertainty, with excessive checking. These individuals lay great store by punctuality and tidiness and are scrupulous and rigid in outlook. Many of these traits are valuable in clerical work, librarianship and accountancy. Their inflexibility makes them difficult colleagues and employers and their polite, conventional exterior often conceals much hostility. Frequently associated with migraine, dyspepsia and depression, as well as with obsessional neurosis.

Anxious

'Born worriers' whose level of anxiety is always above average and who worry excessively about trivia that do not worry others. Timid, diffident and indecisive. Often worry about health and make frequent visits to doctors' surgeries for reassurance.

Psychopathic

Alternatively antisocial or sociopathic personality. These labels are applied to individuals who behave in a seriously antisocial way, show a wide range of antisocial behaviour from an early age, and are unable to learn from experience or punishment. The central personality defects seem to be an inability to love and empathise with others and an inability to feel guilt. They are usually impulsive, irresponsible and aggressive. Their lack of feeling for others and their cold callous personality sets them apart from other criminals and delinquents, who readily recognise them as abnormal. Often accompanying neurotic symptoms, history of parasuicide, family history of antisocial behaviour and alcoholism. Nearly always antisocial behaviour in childhood with episodes of truancy, serious disobedience and theft. Most show late maturation of personality and improvement in behaviour between the ages of 30 and 40 years. Only a minority of aggressive criminals and murderers fall into this category.

Psychopathic personalities are sometimes divided into two groups — the *aggressive*, described above and the *inadequate*, a group with the same personality defects, leading a feckless life, often abusing alcohol or drugs, but not aggressive or dangerous.

FURTHER READING

Lewis A 1974 Psychopathic personality: a most elusive category. Psychological Medicine 4: 133

10

The psychoneuroses

Psychoneurotic disorders, commonly referred to as 'nervous' illnesses, are characterised by disturbances of feelings, attitudes and habits severe enough to impair the patient's life or to reduce his efficiency. The symptoms are best understood as manifestations of anxiety or as ineffective ways of dealing with anxiety.

Incidence: high, but difficult to estimate accurately. This group of disorders is probably the commonest single cause of ill health encountered in general practice. Symptoms of anxiety and depression are frequent, hysterical and obsessional symptoms less so.

Classification. The psychoneuroses are classified by the symptoms. Overlap occurs between the various subdivisions and many mixed types of psychoneurosis occur, e.g. anxiety and hysterical symptoms may co-exist.

Anxiety neurosis

Anxiety is a fundamental mode of response experienced by everyone. It is analogous to pain in that both serve as a warning to the organism. In psychoneurosis anxiety appears inappropriate to the situation or excessive in degree.

In anxiety neurosis patients show signs of increased autonomic activity, both sympathetic and parasympathetic. There are feelings of tension, concern, apprehension, difficulty in concentrating and insomnia, combined with palpitations, sweating, gastric disturbance, restlessness, tremulousness, 'tension headache', diarrhoea. The symptoms may be persistent or take the form of acute attacks of anxiety lasting a few minutes or several hours. Depressive symptoms or symptoms of fatigue ('neurasthenia') are often associated with anxiety.

Acute anxiety states occurring in previously stable personalities are usually short-lived and have a good prognosis. Chronic and recurrent anxiety states are found in *anxious personalities,* who have always been timid, diffident, indecisive, fearful and worrying.

Phobic states

A phobia is an unreasonable fear, out of proportion to the situation, which cannot be voluntarily controlled and which leads to avoidance of the object or feared situation. Fears may be normal or abnormal, the dividing line often being a question of severity and incapacity, e.g. fears of flying, of spiders, and of heights. Abnormal fears can be divided into fears of external and internal stimuli. Phobias of internal stimuli comprise obsessive phobias (see obsessional neurosis) and illness phobias (hypochondriasis, venereophobia, etc.). Most fears are of external stimuli. Two-thirds show agoraphobia, and the remainder social phobias, or specific phobias, especially of animals.

Agoraphobia ('housebound housewife' syndrome)

Agoraphobia is the commonest phobic disorder, and one of the most common neuroses in women, who make up 75 per cent of patients. Usually begins in young adult life. Literally a fear of the *agora* (the Greek place of assembly or market-place). The patient fears going out alone, social situations, shopping, travelling, and confined spaces, such as cinemas and churches. There is associated general anxiety, panic attacks, feelings of dizziness and unsteadiness, and often depression or depersonalisation. If the condition becomes established and lasts for more than a year it tends to run a chronic fluctuating course. The husband becomes involved in doing a great deal for his wife, and after a time there is considerable secondary gain to the patient. Often agoraphobic patients do well in hospital but relapse rapidly on returning home.

Social phobias

The next most common group of phobias. Again common in young adults and more frequent in women, usually with shy, sensitive personalities. The fear of social situations may be general but often is concerned with one particular social situation — eating or drinking in public, writing or speaking, or using public toilets. There is little general anxiety.

Hysteria

The symptoms of hysteria usually solve a conflict by resolving the associated anxiety. They have a motivation and often a symbolic meaning which is not recognised by the patient and therefore unconscious. In *malingering* the symptoms are feigned, i.e. consciously produced, and the distinction can usually be made without difficulty clinically, although difficult to prove in law. Once established the symptoms may provide gain to the patient.

Features of the hysterical personality (see p. 48) are often present. Hysterical patients have often experienced periods of illness in childhood and have learned the advantages of the *sick role* and *illness behaviour,* i.e. that patient status can be rewarding in gaining sympathy and attention and in avoiding duties and obligations.

Conversion hysteria

The conflict is solved by the development of a somatic symptom, e.g. paralysis, anaesthesia, blindness. The symbolism is often obvious e.g. loss of voice in a bride-to-be. The symptoms are varied and may mimic any physical illness. The patient *thinks* he has a disturbance of function, and the symptom corresponds to his *idea* of what it should be. Diagnosis may be difficult when physical symptoms of organic disease are hysterically prolonged or exaggerated. Physical illness must be excluded, but to make a diagnosis of hysteria it is also necessary to show that the symptom serves a purpose, is meaningful, or produces gain for the patient. When re-examined after some years many patients, confidently diagnosed as hysteria, have developed a variety of organic diseases.

Dissociative reactions

Particular experiences or events are dissociated from consciousness and the patient shows amnesia, a fugue state, somnambulism, or rarely multiple personality. So-called 'hysterical' fits are rare, and usually prove to be temporal lobe seizures. Abnormal movements (torticollis etc.) are rarely hysterical and 'globus hystericus' is organic in 80 per cent of cases. Part of the dissociation in hysterical reactions is illustrated by the hysteric's bland cheerful attitude to the symptoms (*belle indifference*).

Hysterical symptoms are more frequent in primitive populations and gross conversion reactions are now rare in Europe. They are also seen in military settings and in schools where *epidemic hysteria* may occur. Conversion reactions are rare in psychiatric practice but can be found in neurological and orthopaedic clinics.

Briquet's syndrome (St. Louis hysteria)

Named after a 19th century French physician and a group of St. Louis psychiatrists. Occurs in patients with a dramatic or complicated medical history beginning before aged 35 who admit to 25 symptoms covering nine of a check list of ten symptom groups, and which cannot be explained by any other diagnosis. Nearly all women, often a family history, often psychopathic personalities. Defines a group of intensely hypochondriacal and invalid patients — 'thick file cases' — with a poor prognosis.

Munchausen syndrome

After a fictional Baron (1786) who had 'fabulous adventures'. Also called 'peregrinating problem patients' and 'hospital hobos'. These patients spend many years seeking repeated hospital stays, investigations and operations, by accurately feigning disease. Asher originally described three types — laparotomophilia migrans (acute abdominal pain), haemorrhagica histrionica (blood in urine, vomit, stool) and neurologica diabolica (faints, fits, headaches). Others occur. Usually men, starting in twenties. These patients avoid psychiatrists and little is known about their life histories and motivation, but they may begin their hospital careers after a period of physical illness or a major crisis in their lives.

The Ganser syndrome

Hysterical pseudodementia. Described in prisons by Ganser in 1898. Characterised by approximate answers (2 + 2 = 5; a dog has five legs) and clouding of consciousness. Nowadays the syndrome is more often seen in organic states and schizophrenia.

Obsessional neurosis

An *obsession* exists whenever a person cannot exclude thoughts from consciousness, distinguishes them as unreasonable and attempts to resist them but cannot do so. Obsessions occur in many psychiatric conditions, notably in depressive illness and schizophrenia. When they are primary the diagnosis of obsessive compulsive or obsessive ruminative neurosis is made. *Rumination* is the term applied to repetitive obsessional thinking; *compulsions* are acts which the patient feels compelled to carry out. When these acts are stereotyped and repetitive they become rituals. Obsessions with sex, violence, death, dirt, excrement and germs are usual. Washing and checking rituals are common.

Obsessional neurosis is often associated with an *obsessional personality* in which there is a tendency to excessive orderliness, punctuality, scrupulousness and rigidity of behaviour and attitudes.

The incidence of obsessional neurosis is low. Age of onset is usually between 15 and 25. These neuroses, when fully developed, have a poorer prognosis than other neurotic reactions and are resistant to treatment. Clomipramine, orally or by infusion, may be of value. Intensive psychotherapy is rarely indicated but supportive psychotherapy is helpful. In very severe and chronic cases functional neurosurgery is of value and behaviour therapy is also useful.

Post-traumatic neurosis

This type of psychoneurosis is seen in patients who have been subjected to a trauma which has involved a sudden threat to life. Physical injury may or may not occur. Most cases occur after accidents and claims for compensation often complicate diagnosis and treatment to the extent that *accident neurosis* or *compensation neurosis* have been alternative labels for the condition. In *battle neurosis* the strain and exhaustion of combat, with or without a traumatic incident, initiates symptoms.

The symptoms may comprise any of the neurotic symptoms already mentioned but irritability, tension, poor concentration and nightmares, often of a repetitive kind, are common. Motor manifestations, especially tics, may occur.

The prognosis is generally good. Post-traumatic neurosis is common after head injury and these cases have a poorer prognosis, particularly when there is a claim for compensation.

Compensation neurosis is most often found after road traffic and industrial accidents. There is elaboration or prolongation of the symptoms related to the injury and this occurs twice as often as in non-compensation injuries, e.g. sport. More frequent in minor than in major injuries, especially head injuries (see p. 29). More common in unskilled and semi-skilled workers and immigrants, perhaps related to language difficulties. Often previous neurotic history and symptoms may persist after financial settlement' Lengthy legal proceedings and the adversary system in court do nothing to help these cases.

Aetiology of psychoneurosis

Genetic factors are particularly important in anxiety neurosis. In general, there is a 60 per cent concordance in monozygotic twins, 30 per cent in dizygotic.

Learning-theory models of neurosis have been created in animal work using conditioned avoidance responses to mimic phobic symptoms (see p. 110). All animal work is difficult to compare with human neurosis because of their lack of language.

Childhood. Most adult neurotics do *not* have a history of childhood neurosis. Conversely most neurotic children recover.

Family. There is an increase in neurotic symptoms in the spouses of neurotic patients. Probably due to marital interaction and not to selection by assortative mating.

Sociology. Cultural expectations are of more importance in neurosis than in other psychiatric disorders. Once society (doctor, family) has *labelled* a person as sick or deviant it is difficult for him or her not to take up the *sick role* or show *illness behaviour.* These ideas do not account for the initial symptoms but frequently help to explain *secondary deviance*, e.g. elaboration of symptoms, invalidism. Once a patient is labelled as such, he may not be regarded as responsible, may give up behaving responsibly, or may be stigmatised by others, with further secondary effects.

Psychogenesis. The Freudian view is that the causes of neurosis are 'intrapsychic'. Although superficially the symptoms may seem related to current events and stresses they are usually inappropriate or exaggerated responses and can only be explained in terms of past experiences. 'Intrapsychic anxiety may be expressed directly or other neurotic symptoms may develop as *defences* against anxiety. Freud regarded the experience of anxiety, as in simple anxiety neurosis or in nightmares, as a failure of defence or as a signal, alerting the individual to the need for defences against further anxiety.

Hysteria. Was studied by Freud & Breuer (1895), who explained the symptoms as caused by repressed memories (*repression*), the *conversion* of ideas into bodily symptoms, and *dissociation* of mental processes (as in fugue states). The symptom can be viewed as a symbolic representation of a conflict in that it combines the expression of a wish with the arousal of defences against that wish (e.g. desire to run away from battle and fear of being thought a coward 'solved' by hysterical paralysis of the legs).

Obsessional neurosis. The symptoms represent defences against instinctual impulses, often of an aggressive nature. Guilt arises from these impulses with ambivalence towards parental figures. The rituals are seen as attempts to *undo* the guilt. The neurotic shows in an exaggerated and distorted form the characteristics of the obsessional personality (anal-erotic character), namely the need to achieve security by arranging the environment in an orderly, regular fashion. Freud regarded the neurosis as a regression to the anal-erotic phase. The *obsessions* are seen as repressed wishes, unacceptable to the patient and felt by him to be foreign; thought is isolated from feeling.

Phobic states (called anxiety hysteria by Freud) are also regarded as defences. The object of the fear is thought to be unimportant in itself and to be a *symbol* of some impulse or wish that the patient cannot face. Phobic patients deal with anxiety by avoiding it and any conflict that may lead to it.

Treatment and prognosis

Psychotherapy, behaviour therapy and minor tranquillisers all have applications in the management and the appropriate treatment chapters deal with them at length. Detailed history taking is the initial step and itself institutes treatment. Mild and recent symptoms require only simple treatment and carry a good prognosis. Severe symptoms require more intensive and time consuming methods. Longstanding symptoms have a poor prognosis. Of the neuroses seen in general practice some two-thirds will remit spontaneously within a year.

FURTHER READING

Blackwell B 1968 The Munchausen syndrome. British Journal of Hospital Medicine 1: 98-102

Chodoff P 1974 The diagnosis of hysteria: an overview. American Journal of Psychiatry 131: 1013-1018

Kraüpl-Taylor F 1979 Psychopathology. Butterworths, London

Miner G D 1973 The evidence for genetic components in the neuroses. Arch gen Psychiat 29: 111-118

Whitlock F A 1967 The Ganser syndrome. British Journal of Psychiatry 113: 19-29

11

Alcoholism

The World Health Organisation attempted to define alcoholics as 'those excessive drinkers whose dependence on alcohol has attained such a degree that it causes a noticeable mental disturbance or an interference with their bodily and mental health, their interpersonal relations and their smooth social and economic functioning'.

This is a social rather than a medical definition and depends on social and cultural factors which may vary, e.g. excessive for whom, when, compared with what other group, in what culture? It is generally agreed that alcoholism is a *dependency disorder* in which the alcoholic shows both psychological and physical dependence. Physical dependence implies that withdrawal leads to a characteristic syndrome, and this holds true for established drinking. It can easily be seen how psychological dependence, produced by the anxiety-relieving effects of alcohol, can in time lead to physical dependence.

Normal drinking
A single whisky, a half-pint of beer and a large glass of table wine each contain about 8 grams of alcohol. It is useful to think of this as an *alcohol unit*. The effects and stages of acute intoxication are well known. 'Cheery' equals 80 mg/ml blood levels, 'merry' equals 100 mg/ml, and 'unsteady' equals 140 mg/ml. These levels can be attained in one hour by drinking 4, 5 and 6 units respectively.

In Scotland 30 per cent of all the alcohol consumed is drunk by 3 per cent of the population: the *heavy drinkers*, mostly male manual workers under 30 years. This group drinks over two bottles of whisky weekly or its equivalent; they are heavy smokers, often have heavy drinking fathers and do not see themselves as heavy drinkers. This 'at risk' group is in danger of becoming dependent if a *critical dose* is exceeded. Estimates of the critical dose vary; it is in the region of 16 units daily for several months, i.e., seven to eight pints of beer, half a bottle of spirits or two bottles of wine daily.

Aetiology

A plausible theory must explain why the majority of the population drinks alcohol but only a minority becomes dependent. It must also explain other known facts about alcoholism. Male cases outnumber women by at least five to one. Many are single, and the peak age of presentation is from 40 to 50 years. It is more common at the extremes of social class. There are racial and cultural differences: Scots outnumber English, Catholics usually outnumber Jews, and blacks outnumber whites in the U.S.A. Rural rates are higher than urban, and those in the drink trade or involved in business entertaining have higher rates. The sons of alcoholics have twice the normal risk.

Much research — genetic, social, metabolic, endocrine, and psychological — has yielded no convincing results. Learning theory offers a simple theory of the development of alcoholism in terms of operant conditioning; immediate rewards (relief) are more effective than delayed punishment (hangover). Later, non-reward factors (fear of withdrawal symptoms) may reinforce continued drinking.

Prevalence

Prevalence is about 1 per cent in Britain, but concealment and denial make accurate figures impossible to obtain. First admission rates for alcoholism underestimate the problem. Jellinek devised a formula for estimating prevalence from deaths due to alcoholic cirrhosis which proved reasonably accurate. Consumption of spirits, beer and wine is rising in Britain, and alcoholism is also rising, especially in younger males.

Admissions for alcoholism in Scotland have increased sixfold in the last 20 years. Among male admissions alcoholism is twice as common as any other diagnosis. Convictions for drunkenness have doubled in only six years. These increases are paralleled by a steady rise in the whole population's consumption of alcohol in Britain and other European countries over the last 20 years. A correlation has been established between this rise, rising admission rates, and the rising mortality from liver cirrhosis. The *Ledermann hypothesis* claims that there is a fixed relation between average and excessive consumption of alcohol. If a critical or harmful level of alcohol intake is established then the 'at risk' population can be calculated from the average consumption of the population. Further, if the average consumption rises or falls there will be corresponding changes in the 'at risk' population. If a population as a whole drinks less it will have fewer alcohol problems, and *vice versa*.

Types

1. Loss of control. Bout drinking; one drink triggers off a binge. Usually spirits. Commonest in Britain and North America.

2. Inability to abstain. Constant daily drinking, usually of wine or beer. Common in Italy and France.

Stages

1. Symptomatic pre-dependent.

2. Prodromal. The drinker avoids discussing his consumption, begins secret drinking, minimises amount, feels guilty, and may have amnesia for the previous night's drinking (alcoholic palimpsests).

3. Dependency. Psychological and physical — withdrawal signs if stops.

4. Chronic. Social deterioration, physical and psychiatric complications.

Diagnosis

Many alcoholics deny difficulties and are brought reluctantly by relatives. They may agree that they have a drinking problem but argue about the label of alcoholism, which should be avoided. Enquire about work and domestic problems, withdrawal symptoms, amnesia, morning shakiness, nausea. Obtain account from relative.

Complications

Social

By the time the alcoholic is willing to accept help these are almost inevitable. Frequent changes of job or unemployment, unhappy marriage or divorce, financial and housing problems, multiple and complicated financial difficulties.

Physical

1. Acute intoxication, coma, etc.

2. Withdrawal syndromes: the 'shakes', delirium tremens.

3. Deficiency and nutritional syndromes: peripheral neuropathy, Korsakoff's psychosis, Wernicke's encephalopathy (confusion, ataxia, eye signs — nystagmus, rectus palsy).

4. Epilepsy: common at various stages of alcoholism, especially during withdrawal.

5. Other complications include myopathies, cardiac disease, cirrhosis, pancreatic disease, malabsorption disorders, hypoglycaemia, hyperlipaemia, magnesium deficiency.

Psychiatric

1. Alcoholic hallucinosis
2. Alcoholic paranoid state — often 'morbid jealousy syndrome'
3. Alcoholic dysmnesic states
4. Alcoholic dementia
5. Suicide.

Treatment and prognosis

Prognosis is poor; even those who do well usually have initial relapses. At best one-third remain abstinent after treatment, even of carefully selected patients. There is no evidence that lengthy admissions are better than short ones, or that admission is superior to out-patient treatment except for brief 'drying out'. Sedatives and psychotropic drugs are best avoided except to cover withdrawal, as they are often abused. Treatments include Antabuse (disulfiram) and Abstem (citrated calcium carbide), which produce an unpleasant or dangerous reaction if alcohol is taken; and aversion therapy with apomorphine or electric shock aimed at producing a conditioned response (vomiting or pain) to alcohol. These physical methods are falling into disuse. Group techniques are used by psychiatrists and in Alcoholics Anonymous; the latter's results are better. In recent years there has been a vogue for teaching alcoholics to drink normally (controlled drinking) but AA and the majority of doctors reject this approach and regard it as a counsel of despair.

Detoxification ('drying out') centres and after-care hostels are being developed. National and Regional Councils for Alcoholism have established advice centres and have encouraged health education programmes to detect alcohol problems at an early stage.

Understandably, the alcoholic meets much distrust and prejudice during rehabilitation. The drinker who rejects help earlier often accepts it when his condition has deteriorated. Many doctors fail to diagnose alcohol problems in the early stages or reject them by taking up a moralistic attitude.

Most therapeutic hope lies in prophylaxis. Energetic efforts are now being made to offer help to the 'at risk' population of young male heavy drinkers and to educate the public in normal drinking and safe limits. The political problem is to reduce average consumption, most simply solved by increasing taxation and restricting opening hours, but unpopular with both public and politicians. In terms of average income the cost of spirits has halved in the last 20 years.

FURTHER READING

Clare A W 1979 The causes of alcoholism. British Journal of Hospital Medicine (April): 403-411
Dight S E 1976 Scottish drinking habits. HMSO, London
Edwards G, Gross M M 1976 Alcohol dependence: provisional description of a syndrome. British Medical Journal 1: 1058-1061
Kessel N, Walton H 1969 Alcoholism. Penguin, Harmondsworth
Kendell R E 1979 Alcoholism: a medical or a political problem. British Medical Journal 1: 367-371
Madden J S 1979 A guide to alcohol and drug dependence. Wright, Bristol
Royal College of Psychiatrists 1979 Alcohol and alcoholism

12

Drug dependence

The World Health Organisation has defined drug dependence as a 'state of periodic or chronic intoxication, detrimental to the individual and to society, produced by the repeated consumption of the drug. Its characteristics include: an overpowering desire or need to continue taking the drug and to obtain it by any means; a tendency to increase the dose; psychic and sometimes physical dependence on the effects of the drug.'

For many years dependence on dangerous drugs was rare in the United Kingdom and occurred mainly in professional workers with access to drugs (e.g. doctors, pharmacists, nurses) or was iatrogenic, following the prescription of powerful analgesics post-operatively or in chronic physical illness. These cases have been overshadowed in the last twenty years by an alarming increase in addiction in young people. Drugs used by addicts include morphine, cocaine, synthetic analgesics (pethidine, physeptone), barbiturates and amphetamines. The use of cannabis (marihuana, hashish) is increasing among young people but its status as a true drug of addiction and as a precursor of abuse of 'hard' drugs is debatable.

In the U.K. there has been a recent tendency for multiple drug abuse to occur. Drug abuse by younger people has to be viewed against a background of serious alcohol abuse in society and the still widespread use of tobacco by adults.

Morphine, heroin (Di-acetyl-morphine)
Subcutaneous ('skin-pop') and intravenous ('main-line') routes are used. Nausea, sweating and malaise occur before pleasurable 'honeymoon stage'. Light sleep and wakefulness alternate allowing the 'opium dreams' to occur. Constipation and pupillary contraction are found. Appetite is poor and libido is reduced. Abstinence syndrome occurs 9-12 hours after withdrawal — perspiration, yawning, restlessness, insomnia, rhinorrhoea, rigor, diarrhoea and cramps.

Cocaine
Uncommon by itself but often taken with other drugs to increase libido. Drugs are sniffed in 'decks' with the risk of nasal septal perforation, or are taken by 'main-line'. Initial alertness and increased energy are often followed by collapse, cramps, twitching, delirium or toxic psychosis. Formication (tactile hallucinations) occurs.

Pethidine
Highest incidence in doctors and nurses who may take it for relief of pain (e.g. dysmenorrhoea). Muscular twitching, tremor, dilated pupils, confusion and fits may be found. EEG changes occur.

Barbiturates
Common in United States of America and Western Europe. May alternate with amphetamine taking. Severe dependence when about 0.8g or more are taken each day. Confusion and ataxia or nystagmus is common and may simulate dementia, drunkenness or neurological lesion. Abrupt withdrawal usually produces convulsions. Withdrawal symptoms are anxiety, headache, tremor, vomiting and weakness. Recent campaigns have urged doctors to severely limit the prescription of these drugs.

Amphetamines
Commenced with the prescription of this and related drugs (e.g. phenmetrazine) to curb appetite. Initial stimulation is followed by toxic effects of the drug and paranoid psychosis mimicking schizophrenia may be seen. Main withdrawal symptom is depression. Most doctors have agreed to ban prescription of amphetamine and related drugs.

Lysergic acid diethylamide 25 (LSD 25, 'Acid')
May be used to produce hallucinations and pseudomystical experiences. Danger of precipitating schizophrenia-like psychosis. True addiction unlikely.

Cannabis, marihuana
World wide increase in use of this drug (grass, pot, ganja, reefer, hash, etc.) by younger people. Feared by some authorities as leading to other drugs ('escalation') but occasional use is relatively safe. Drug is illegal in most countries and may be used as part of protest against authority.

In North America a policy of 'decriminalising' cannabis reduces the penalty for possession of small amounts for personal use. Effects erratic but usually dreamy, tranquil state, increased auditory sensibility, sexual excitement. Not unlike effects of alcohol. Dangerous when driving.

Glue sniffing

A number of organic solvents are abused by young people, often the very young. All are potentially dangerous and permanent damage to the brain, liver and kidney may result.

Aspirin

Aspirin and other readily available analgesics are widely consumed. Middle aged and neurotic women are particularly prone to abuse aspirin. Renal damage may occur (phenacetin now withdrawn). Also risk of gastrointestinal bleeding.

Treatment

The Dangerous Drugs Regulations, 1968 lay down that heroin and cocaine, apart from their analgesic use, may be prescribed only by doctors specially licensed by the Home Secretary. In practice such doctors are usually hospital consultants who treat heroin addiction. The Government has powers to introduce further regulations limiting prescribing of dangerous drugs at any time it may prove necessary. There is a statutory requirement for any doctor seeing an addict to send written particulars to the Home Office within seven days. Licences are only valid for prescribing at a named hospital, such departments becoming 'special centres'.

These regulations were designed to make heroin available to registered addicts and minimise the growth of a 'black-market'. The lack of compulsion means that many addicts seek maintenance supplies rather than cure. For withdrawal admission to hospital is essential and methadone and chlorpromazine are used. Extensive psychotherapy and rehabilitation are essential. The mortality from intercurrent infection among addicts, e.g. serum hepatitis, septicaemia, is high and the prognosis poor.

Much of the drug abuse does not come to medical attention but many young 'users' have psychological or personality problems and refuse medical and social help.

FURTHER READING

Logan F (ed) 1979 Cannabis. Quartermaine House

13

Disorders of sex and reproduction

Because of the attitudes of society and of individuals it is only in recent years that it has been possible to build up an adequate body of knowledge of human sexual behaviour. Paradoxically, more is known about sexual deviations than about normal sexuality.

To deal with the sexual problems brought by patients the doctor should be able to relate them to available systematic knowledge rather than to his own prejudices, moral attitudes and limited personal experience. Ethical and religious considerations are involved in sexual behaviour and should always be respected. The doctor's task is to understand and not to pass judgement.

In all animals sexual drives stem from the reproductive instinct but in humans, because of the long period of maturation, the emotional concomitants are of particular importance. Physical sexual maturity is reached in adolescence. Psychosexual maturity, involving stable sexual adjustment and stable and lasting emotional relationships is only reached later and in a few people it is never fully attained.

The child's attitude to his parents and his emotional relationships with them have an important effect in determining adult sexual behaviour, e.g. the young man tends to choose girl-friends according to the ideas of femininity which he has built up from his contacts with his mother. The Freudian theory of infantile sexuality, culminating in the 'Oedipal situation', lays particular stress on these factors in personality and psychosexual development.

Adolescence
Sexual problems are universal at this time and medical advice is often sought. The adolescent though sexually mature is psychologically immature and unable to take on adult responsibilities, at least in Western civilisation. The resulting conflict leads to anxiety and a search for sexual outlets.

Masturbation as an outlet for adolescents is normal. Guilt feelings are often aroused, however, and are fostered by folklore and rumours suggesting that masturbation does physical, mental and moral damage. With psychosexual maturity and heterosexual activity, masturbation is reduced.

Homosexual behaviour, i.e. sexual activities between members of the same sex, is common in adolescents, especially in closed communities such as public schools and service camps. It usually represents a transitory phase and disappears with maturity. Again guilt feelings and emotional distress are common.

Emotional identifications ('crushes', hero-worship and calf-love, etc.) are common, especially in girls. These frustrated, intense, but short-lived identifications with older people — pop stars, teachers, etc. — may be a source of distress to the adolescent.

Sexual dysfunction in men

In males there are three types of potency disorder: impotence, failure to ejaculate, and premature ejaculation. *Acute onset impotence* occurs in young males, is associated with anxiety, and usually has a definite physical or psychological precipitant. These men usually seek help spontaneously. They do not lose the capacity to respond erotically, retain morning erections, and can masturbate. *Insidious onset impotence* usually begins over the age of 30. There is a gradual onset with no clear precipitant. The man seeks help only at his wife's request. There is a general loss of libido and erotic response. Anxiety is secondary, most often provoked by the complaints of the spouse. Ejaculatory failure may be an early symptom in this group. *Premature ejaculation* is a separate syndrome, not associated with impotence. It has usually been present since puberty, and is found in tense anxious individuals.

Treatment

The treatment of sexual disorders has advanced in recent years using behavioural techniques. Couples are treated together, often by a male and female therapist, with various techniques introduced by Masters and Johnson. Apart from relaxation and re-education these include *sensate focus*, in which the couple caress each other, but do not attempt coitus; the emphasis is on experiencing and giving pleasure and on avoiding the anxiety of performing. There is a graded progression to orgasm and the treatment is similar to systematic desensitisation. In premature ejaculation this is combined with the 'squeeze technique', the female partner squeezing the glans penis firmly to prevent ejaculation.

Sexual dysfunction in women

Ranges from temporary lack of interest in coitus and failure to experience orgasm to active distaste and fear (diffuse sexual phobia).

Vaginismus is a conditioned muscular spasm of the muscles around the vaginal introitus; dyspareunia describes pain on penetration — neither are related to ability to experience orgasm. As in the male there is wide individual variation in female sexual response. Not all women invariably experience orgasm yet many now expect to do so and seek advice if they do not. The menstrual cycle, childbirth and age all have effects on libido. Psychogenic causes of frigidity are much more common than physical or anatomical problems, but the latter must be excluded. In severe cases with non-consummation ('virgin wives'), a disturbed relationship with the father is usual and the woman often has an hysterical personality.

Treatment results vary and are poor if the marital relationship in general is disturbed and if neurotic symptoms co-exist. Vaginismus is successfully treated with relaxation and graded dilators. Sensate focus techniques and the use of electric vibrators are useful in anorgasmia. The couples' motivation, which may be difficult to determine at first, is important in determining outcome. Psychotherapy is indicated in some cases.

Sexual anomalies
Homosexuality, exhibitionism, transvestism, fetishism and sado-masochism fall under this heading. In each case the dividing line between normality and abnormality may be hard to draw; the division is partly social and varies in different cultures.

Homosexuality
The most frequent deviation. Common in adolescence and in all-male communities (facultative homosexuality). It is found in many immature mammals and in all human cultures, in some of which it evokes no social disapproval or legal restraint. Probably one-third of the male population have had some homosexual experience at some time in their lives, but only about four per cent are exclusively homosexual. Bisexuality is common. The aetiology is unknown. Genetic factors are of doubtful significance. Hormone studies show no differences in testosterone levels although perinatal androgen deficiency has been suggested. Nuclear sex is normal. In some cases psychogenic factors can be seen, e.g. disturbed parent–child relationship, or seduction and traumatic experiences in childhood. The latter accounts for severe legal penalties for offences against those under 16. Since the Sexual Offences Act 1967 homosexual acts between men over 21 in private have been legal.

Homosexuals usually have brief affairs and are often promiscuous. Activities include mutual masturbation, fellatio and anal intercourse.

Because of their status as a minority they have an increased tendency to depression and suicide. They are not often effeminate and have no particular personality traits.

Female homosexuality (Lesbianism — from Sappho's island, Lesbos) also has a frequency of about 4 per cent. Close friendships and physical displays of affection between women are more acceptable socially. Most Lesbians are bisexual, many married. They are less promiscuous than male homosexuals and have more lasting affairs. Also subject to depression. Disturbed family background usual.

Other deviations

Paedophilia: Erotic attraction to pre-pubertal children. Homosexual paedophiliacs form a distinct group from other homosexuals.

Sadism: Taking sexual pleasure in cruelty. Named after the Marquis de Sade, (1740-1814) author of *Justine*.

Masochism is sexual pleasure derived from experiencing cruelty or humiliation, after Leopold von Sacher-Masoch, 19th century author of *Venus in Furs*. Often co-exist — sado-masochism. Very common in male fantasy and catered for by pornography (Sady May'), but sadistic acts, including sexual murder, are very rare.

Fetishism: Male deviation in which a specific object or material becomes the focus of sexual interest (rubber, leather, foot and shoe, hair, etc). Rarely comes to medical attention.

Voyeurism: 'Peeping Toms' who derive sexual satisfaction by looking. Akin to *exhibitionism* — indecent exposure — display of genitals and/or masturbation. Usually quiet, impotent men who are not dangerous.

Transvestism: Cross dressing, wearing 'drag'. May be associated with fetishism or homosexuality, but usually exists alone.

Transexualism: Very rare, occurs in both sexes. Transexuals believe and feel that they 'really' belong to the opposite sex and find their existing genitals repugnant. They have felt like this from an early age and have a strong need to change their sex, persistently demanding surgery. There are no abnormalities of anatomy, hormone, endocrine functions or of genital or chromosomal sex. The problem is one of psychosexual identity. Surgical and hormonal treatment of males who have been living successfully as females gives acceptable results.

Treatment. Many deviants never seek treatment or are seen by the psychiatrist only when legal offences have been committed. Such cases, without adequate motivation for treatment, can rarely be helped. Some patients present with symptoms (anxiety, depression) which mask or obscure the fundamental difficulties. Others (usually young adults) may seek help directly in the solution of their psychosexual difficulties.

Each case must be considered in the light of the circumstances of the referral, the history, the patient's attitude to his anomaly and the nature and severity of any associated psychiatric condition.

Stilboestrol in large doses may be used to suppress libido temporarily. Psychotherapy, in suitable cases, may deal with the psychosexual problems, or help the patient to live with his anomaly without clashing with society. Aversion by behaviour therapy techniques may be useful in selected cases. Complete cure is infrequent.

Termination of pregnancy

Since the Abortion Act, 1968 (see p. 103) large numbers of pregnancies have been terminated on 'mental health' grounds. Doctors vary widely in their interpretation of the social and psychiatric spirit of the Act, but there has been an increasing tendency, in face of changing public opinion, to provide abortion on demand. It can be argued that there are few or no psychiatric grounds for termination — the severely mental subnormal and the chronically schizophrenic do not suffer a deterioration in health through pregnancy, and the fact that they would be unable to care for the child is not legal ground for termination. Conversely it has been argued by other psychiatrists that continuing an unwanted pregnancy will always have adverse effects on the mental health of the mother.

Extensive follow-up studies since the Act show that very few women who have had terminations experience severe remorse or depression as a result, regardless of religious affiliation. Equally, in those refused, no serious mental illness occurs, although unhappiness and social distress may result and the unwanted children may suffer subsequently.

Puerperal illnesses

Psychosis

Prevalence — 1 in 1000 births. Not an entity and classified as affective, schizophrenic, etc., rather than 'puerperal psychosis'. Patient usually well for first few days post-partum; 60 per cent begin in first month, 80 per cent within three months. Only 1 per cent organic, remainder affective or schizophrenic. Often atypical symptoms in first week, with some clouding of consciousness. Differential diagnosis: puerperal cerebral thrombo-phlebitis, distinguished by neurological signs.

Treatment and prognosis as for other affective and schizophrenic illnesses. Risk of recurrence in future pregnancies is one in five, i.e. more than 100 times the post-partum risk in general population.

Neurosis

Most mothers experience transient weepiness and poor concentration in the week after delivery (post-partum blues). Neurotic depression is common in the first year, usually after the first child in young, anxious women, often of below average intelligence and over-dependent on their own mothers. They show anxiety, depression and have difficulty in coping with the baby.

Most psychiatric units provide facilities for admitting mothers and babies, and find them helpful in treating both psychoses and neuroses in the puerperium.

Menstruation and the menopause

A subject surrounded by myth. Many women are tense and irritable premenstrually, and female suicides are more frequent at this time. Whatever the psychiatric symptom, it tends to be worse before and during menstruation. In those cases with fluid retention — the premenstrual syndrome — diuretics and hormonal treatment may be helpful.

Psychiatric symptoms increase just before and during the year of the menopause; immediately afterwards they decrease. In contrast vasomotor symptoms (hot flushes, etc.) occur in the five years after the menopause. It is likely that psychiatric symptoms at this time are psychogenic rather than caused by hormonal changes. Many women are influenced by superstitions about the 'change' and are at a time of life when they have to abandon their maternal role: if they have little to substitute for it, depression and anxiety result. Depressive symptoms are especially common after hysterectomy.

FURTHER READING

Bancroft J 1974 Deviant sexual behaviour — modification and assessment. OUP, Oxford
Gillan P 1978 Treatment of sexual dysfunctions in Gaind R N and Hudson B L: current themes in psychiatry. Macmillan, London
Kaplan H S 1978 The new sex therapy: active treatment of sexual dysfunctions. Penguin, Harmondsworth
Williams A H 1975 Problems of homosexuality. British Medical Journal 3: 426-428

14

Psychiatry and physical illness

Liaison psychiatry
Physical and psychiatric illness coexist more than should occur by
chance, because stress and life events may precipitate both. 25 per cent
of attenders at medical outpatient clinics have psychiatric disorder,
mostly mild affective illness. The increasing number of psychiatric
units in general hospitals and perhaps the increased specialisation of
physicians and surgeons has given the psychiatrist a useful role in their
wards and clinics. Psychiatric disorder is notably frequent in
gynaecological and gastrointestinal clinics — up to 50 per cent in the
latter. Apart from assessing self poisonings and diagnosing the causes
of disturbed behaviour the psychiatrist has often to facilitate
communication between patients and staff and even between staff
members. All physical illnesses have psychological consequences,
many have psychological precipitants, and a few psychological causes.
All these can be of diagnostic, prognostic and therapeutic importance.
This *psychosomatic* approach has always been part of the competent
doctor's technique.

Psychological response to physical illness
All physical illness has psychological *effects*. The woman who
discovers a lump in her breast or the man who survives a myocardial
infarction may react in various ways. These patterns of response can
be healthy or unhealthy. *Anxiety* and *depression* are obvious and
common responses, but can vary greatly in degree and
appropriateness. *Denial* of the illness or its gravity may occur, as can
preoccupation. In convalescence, *prolongation of the sick role* may lead
to *invalidism*. These patterns vary with the type of illness, the patient's
personality and his social background. All must be dealt with in
successful rehabilitation. The same physical disability, be it hemiplegia, blindness or severe rheumatoid arthritis, will lead to
permanent invalidism in some and be completely transcended by
others. Increasing recognition of these factors leads to early attention
to them in rehabilitation.

Physical illness in psychiatric patients

Patients presenting with mainly psychological symptoms often have causative, contributory or associated physical illness. Depression may be an early symptom of malignant disease in middle-aged men. Diabetes, vitamin B12 deficiency, frontal meningiomas and thyroid disease are all easily missed. Surveys of patients attending psychiatric out-patient clinics reveal physical illness in a third of cases. Of these illnesses half are 'causative'. There is a place both for routine physical examination and a small battery of laboratory screening tests in the initial investigation of all psychiatric patients.

Psychosomatic medicine

Psychosomatic medicine can mean: a) a *holistic* approach to patients, considering the interaction of social, psychological and physical factors in each patient. This is the accepted usage today; b) a more limited view restricting the term to diseases in which stress or emotion may produce physical changes in organs supplied by the autonomic nervous system, and in which certain types of personality are associated with particular diseases.

Several diseases fall into this last category; migraine, peptic ulcer, irritable bowel syndrome and asthma are generally accepted as examples. In the heyday of psychosomatic medicine, psychological factors were thought to be causative in these conditions. They are now seen as contributory, precipitating and aggravating. They may operate through long-continued stress or through an accumulation of stressful life events before the onset of the illness. For example, migraine attacks are often related to periods of stress or repressed hostility, but typically the attack occurs only when the situation is past and the stress is over — 'week-end migraine'. The patient with migraine tends to be intelligent, and to show obsessional personality traits (persistent, orderly, thorough).

The best known study on such factors in a particular disease is Friedman and Rosenman's work on 'Type A' behaviour in coronary artery disease. In a large U.S. male sample they studied risk factors and isolated a pattern of competitiveness, aggression, hostility, exaggerated time urgency, with dependability, self-control and industriousness. Such behaviour was associated with increased rates of ischaemic heart disease and was related to raised lipid and cholesterol levels. This personality factor was only one among others — smoking, hypertension, family history, etc. and illustrates the important but restricted role of psychological factors in disease.

Myocardial infarction affords other examples. In the week or two after infarction up to 30 per cent of patients are found to show significant psychological disturbance; its onset in some preceding the event. Many will have had an increase in stressful life events before the episode. If the psychological aspects of rehabilitation are neglected (e.g. advice on exercise, return to work, sexual activity) then invalidism will be much higher than it need be.

In such medical cases the psychiatrist's only expertise may be the time and ability to take a full history covering social, emotional and personality factors. Information of use in management is often revealed.

Psychophysiology and stress

Early work was carried out by Cannon (1871-1945) who related physiological responses to emotions and explained them as 'fight or flight' reactions. Wolf & Wolff in their classical experiments on Tom's gastric fistula were able to relate gastric vascularity and secretion directly to emotional change.

More recently the neurophysiological and neuroendocrine pathways by which acute stress affects the body have been well established. Hypothalamic lesions in animals produce gastrointestinal disorders. In animal experiments, restraint or avoidance of electric shock can produce gastric ulcers and other gastrointestinal disorders. The significance of the animal's 'helplessness' is relevant in such experiments.

Animal experiments also show that autonomic responses such as heart-rate and blood pressure can be altered by reinforcement. These findings led to the use of biofeedback techniques in humans, in which autonomic changes are displayed to the subject who can then monitor or control the changes, e.g. by relaxation. Biofeedback techniques are being used in patients suffering from a wide range of disorders such as hypertension, migraine and torticollis.

Selye's explanation of stress as a general reaction which, with prolonged exposure, can lead to exhaustion, allows the findings from animal studies involving acute stress to be applied to chronic stress which may be a causative factor in some disorders.

The effects of severe sustained stress have been studied in the survivors of concentration camps and prisoners of war. Such groups, apart from psychiatric sequelae, show an increase in dyspepsia and peptic ulceration, and have a higher mortality from many causes.

There is evidence from the study of life events in relation to illness that significant *clusters* of illness may occur in individuals after periods of increased stress.

Bereavement

Of the normal life stresses to which the individual is exposed, bereavement is usually rated the most severe and will frequently lead to the bereaved person seeking medical help.

Acute grief typically lasts for six to twelve weeks, but significant disturbance persists for one to two years. The first phase, lasting up to two weeks after the death, is of protective numbness, with dissociation and depersonalisation. The bereaved person in this state may cope very adequately with funeral arrangements and outwardly appear surprisingly unmoved, or 'shocked'. This is succeeded by intense grief and distress, with restlessness, attacks of sighing and choking sensations. Over the first three months this gradually gives way to constant depression of variable degree. There is difficulty in communicating and vivid dreams of the dead person and illusions of the dead person's presence occur.

Recognition of this reaction is important for several reasons:

1. Death tends increasingly to be a taboo topic, to the extent that bereaved people are stigmatised. Little allowance is made for the normal process of mourning to take place.

2. It must be distinguished from atypical grief, where the reaction is not only unduly severe or prolonged, but is often characterised by excessive guilt and self-blame, hypochondriasis, and suicidal ideas.

3. The period of bereavement carries a high morbidity and mortality, not only from suicide. Comparison with control groups shows that in the year after a death the bereaved (particularly widowers) consult their doctor more often, are prescribed more drugs, have higher suicide rates and have higher death rates from other causes.

Death and dying

Increasingly, deaths take place in hospital and not at home. This and the decline of religion means that medical and nursing staff are more often asked for help with the psychological problems of those facing death and their relatives. The dying patient's reactions cannot be predicted from his previous personality. The reactions described include acceptance, denial, defiance, depression and bargaining. There are no easy guide lines and there are difficult ethical problems in deciding whether or not to tell the patient he is dying — to have a conspiracy of silence, or to encourage free discussion.

Deafness

Depression is a common reaction to the onset of severe deafness in adult life. In patients with late paraphrenia there is some hearing impairment in 40 per cent and it is possible that the onset of deafness in early adult life or middle age predisposes to ideas of reference and auditory hallucinations. Those who are profoundly deaf from birth or childhood are severely handicapped in many respects: the difficulties in communication and language development have profound psychological effects and there is often a danger that mental handicap will be diagnosed in error.

Plastic surgery

Psychiatric opinion is often necessary in those seeking plastic surgery for minimal disfigurement. Most applicants are young, over-concerned about prominent ears or noses and have sensitive, insecure personalities. Such complaints are known as *dysmorphophobia*. Often the person has been teased or given a nickname in childhood. Although the psychological disturbance may often seem much worse than the deformity, many of these patients do well with surgery. A small minority are psychotic or will become so and can usually be screened out before surgery.

Pain

Laboratory studies on animals and humans have tended to discredit the view of pain as a discrete sensation. In specialist pain clinics, the complex factors which produce the experience of pain for a patient are taken into account. In such settings, the physician has to go beyond the removal or modification of the noxious stimulus and to deal with the patient's characteristic response to pain and his or her interpretation of the pain.

Psychiatric sequelae of medication

Both in liaison psychiatry and in his own practice the psychiatrist often has to consider drugs used for other purposes as causes of psychiatric disorder — iatrogenic illness.

Hypnotics may cause confusional states in the elderly and chronic intoxication when abused. Analgesics may at times lead to confusion, as can sulphonamides, penicillin, and isoniazid.

Hypotensive drugs may cause depression, especially in high doses, and in those predisposed by a previous attack or family history. Reserpine is the worst offender, but methyldopa and guanethidine may also be implicated. In the elderly an excess of digitalis (with or without potassium depletion from an excess of diuretics) may cause confusion and hallucinations.

Cortisone or corticotrophin leads to minor mood change in 40 per cent, major change in 4 per cent — often euphoria and mania.

Oral contraceptives may lead to mild depression in 5-10 per cent, especially with a previous history. Lower with sequential preparations; higher with strongly progestrogenic ones.

Antidepressants can cause hypomania and rarely schizophreniform excitement. Tricyclics can confuse the elderly, as can anti-Parkinson medication. L-dopa often causes mood disturbance or confusion. Amphetamines may cause paranoid psychoses in large doses.

Anticonvulsants may cause slow, apathetic behaviour in large doses.

FURTHER READING

Cooper A F et al 1974 Hearing loss in paranoid and affective psychosis of the elderly. Lancet 2: 851-854

Goldberg D P, Blackwell B 1970 Psychiatric illness in general practice. British Medical Journal 2: 439-443

Hey G G 1970 Psychiatric aspects of cosmetic nasal operation. British Journal of Psychiatry 116: 85-97

Lancet (14 July) 1979 Cost effectiveness of screening tests in psychiatric admissions

Lipowski Z J 1977 Psychosomatic medicine in the seventies: an overview. American Journal of Psychiatry 134: 233-244

Parkes M 1965 Bereavement. Penguin, Harmondsworth

15

Psychiatric problems of old age

The rise in the number of people reaching old age is a major problem for psychiatric services. The proportion over 75 years is the most important. The number in this category is expected to rise by up to 40 per cent in some parts of the U.K. by the year 1991. Mental changes are a part of normal ageing. All old people decline in intellectual power, show narrowing of interest and outlook, are unable to accept new ideas and tend to dwell on the past. Mental illness in old age shows such changes in an exaggerated form. Old people are particularly prone to anxiety and reactive depression precipitated by failing physical health, financial hardship, bereavement, loneliness, lack of self-esteem and social status.

Although elderly people suffer from a wide range of mental illnesses the major problem is that of *senile dementia* and *multi-infarct dementia* (see p. 28). The incidence of dementing illness rises with increasing age. Community surveys suggest that 10 per cent of over 65s need psychiatric help, and after 75 years the figure rises to about 25 per cent. About half of this number have marked or severe dementia. Clearly not every dementing patient can be given hospital admission and there is increasing interest in the organisation of out-patient and community services to help them and their relatives. Elderly people with mental disorder should, ideally, be medically assessed by a psychiatrist and a geriatrician working together. In some areas a joint psychiatric/geriatric assessment unit has been established. The diagnosis of dementia should not be made without full physical examination to exclude possible treatable disorders. *Geriatric psychiatry day hospitals* are able to provide assessment and support for many demented patients and their families.

Where the main problem is that of disturbed behaviour, e.g. wandering, aggressiveness, paranoid delusions, then long term care in a psychiatric hospital may be necessary. Where no special behaviour disorder exists the patient should, if possible, be cared for in a *residential home* provided by the local authority. If there is a significant degree of physical illness as well as mental disorder, long term geriatric care will be required. Many mildly demented elderly people can remain at home provided there is adequate domiciliary support. This can take the form of a home help, home meals service, chiropody, physiotherapy, etc. The *health visitor* or community psychiatric nurse plays a major part in supervising the home care of the elderly. *Voluntary services* also play an increasing part in this branch of psychiatry. Although there is no specific medical treatment for dementia, good care will lengthen the period of time before admission becomes essential. 'Reality Orientation', a form of behaviour therapy (see p. 110), may help to keep the patient in touch with his or her surroundings by intensive retraining in simple skills.

Elderly people also frequently suffer from *affective illness*. This will usually respond to the treatment prescribed for affective illness in younger people. However affective illness in the elderly is frequently associated with co-existing physical illness and every effort should be made to restore the patient to optimum physical health. It is essential to distinguish depression from dementia because of its response to treatment, although the two conditions may coexist. Deafness may precipitate affective and *paranoid illness* in the elderly. Bereavement is a common experience of elderly people and the loss of a spouse, particularly of a wife, is frequently followed by a depressive illness in which social isolation, self neglect, poor nutrition, etc., may eventually lead to the development of a confusional state and admission to a geriatric or psychiatric unit. *Toxic confusional states* are common in elderly people and may be precipitated by quite minor physical illnesses, e.g. urinary tract infection. The excessive use of sedative drugs should also be avoided as these may cause confusion. *Alcohol* abuse is not uncommon in lonely elderly people and may present with a confusional state. *Psychoneurosis* is less often diagnosed in older patients but occurs quite frequently. States of anxiety and reactive depression related to retirement, bereavement, financial difficulty, social isolation and fear of failing physical abilities will require psychological treatment (see Ch. 22).

FURTHER READING

Bromley D B 1977 The psychology of human ageing. Penguin, Harmondsworth
HMSO 1979 Services for the elderly with mental disability in Scotland
Townsend P 1957 The family life of old people. Penguin, Harmondsworth

16

Suicide

Suicide and parasuicide — the more recent and neutral term for attempted suicide — are major topics in current psychiatry, because of the increasing numbers involved and the research they have produced. In the world over 1000 suicides take place daily; in Britain there are over 3000 deaths from suicide annually, and parasuicide is 10 times as common. Self-poisoning now accounts for 15 per cent of all medical admissions, and in patients under 40 years is the commonest cause of admission to hospital medical units.

Suicide is an emotional subject. Several myths are in common circulation: that suicide happens without warning; that those who threaten suicide never do so; that all attempted suicides are attention-seeking and trivial; and that all suicides are mentally ill. All are false. Suicides and parasuicides are two overlapping populations. Suicides tend to be over 45, male, of higher social class and use violent methods; parasuicides tend to be under 45, female, of lower social class, and use self-poisoning.

Parasuicide

The diagnosis in the majority of cases is depression, more often neurotic than endogenous. Many have personality disorders, either immature, or aggressive and antisocial. Many are alcoholics or drug addicts — in a Glasgow study 70 per cent of all self-poisoners had been drinking at the time of the attempt. Self-poisoning is also common in epilepsy, and frequently repeated. Few schizophrenics make attempts. In some cases no formal diagnosis can be made; there is usually a history of an impulsive reaction to acute social distress.

Motives are mixed. Apart from the wish to die, many are seeking aid (the 'Cry for Help'), some are punishing or manipulating family or friends, and some are appealing to fate by gambling with their lives. The *methods* used are increasingly dominated by drugs, particularly barbiturates, aspirin and psychotropic drugs.

Prognosis. After an attempt, 1 in 50 will go on to kill themselves within a year, and in the 10 year period after attempts about 10 per cent will kill themselves and 25 per cent repeat the attempt.

Suicide

Much is known about the general characteristics of groups of suicides. They are predominantly male, old and single, divorced or widowed. They are socially isolated, or have lost status through loss of employment or retirement. Suicide is more common in social classes 1 and 2 and in certain occupations (doctors, dentists and university students). There may be a history of physical illness, commonly painful and chronic, of recent bereavement, or of alcoholism or drug abuse. High rates are linked with high density of population and residence in cities. Frequently there is a history of a broken home in childhood.

Clinically, two main groups of successful suicides can be distinguished. The first have no history of a previous attempt, have stable if dependent previous personalities, and kill themselves without warning, using drastic methods (e.g. hanging, drowning). Often their death is precipitated by bereavement, usually the loss of a spouse. The second have a history of a previous parasuicide. They are often severely disordered personalities, with long histories of poor work records, psychiatric treatment, heavy drinking or criminality. They die from self-poisoning, after warning others, and often with others in the vicinity.

Management

It has been official policy in Britain to have all self-poisonings admitted to hospital examined by a psychiatrist, but it has been shown that properly trained house physicians, nurses and social workers are competent to assess suicidal risk and the need for specialist treatment in these cases.

A simple device for assessing future suicidal risk in a parasuicide is to score one for each of the following items present: antisocial personality, alcohol problem, previous psychiatric admission, previous psychiatric out-patient, previous parasuicide admission, not living with a relative. Those who have no score have less than 5 per cent chance of repetition; those who score 5 to 6 have 50 per cent chance of repetition within five years.

The following check list is made up of items associated with higher suicide rates which should be sought in history taking.

1. Personal and Social:

Male, over 40, widowed, separated or divorced, immigrant, living alone, unemployed or retired, in poor housing.

2. Previous History:

Suicidal attempt, affective disorder, alcoholism, drug abuse.

3. Family History:

Suicide, affective disorder, alcoholism.

4. Personality:

Cyclothymic, psychopathic.

5. Psychiatric disorder:

Affective illness, alcoholism, addiction, early dementia, epilepsy or head injury.

6. Life Stresses:

Bereavement, separation, moving house, loss of job, incapacitating or painful physical illness.

7. Symptoms:

Weight loss, slow speech, insomnia, social withdrawal, loss of interest, hopelessness, self-blame, agitation, suicidal thoughts, physical complications of alcohol.

8. Circumstances of Attempt:

Precautions against discovery, leaving suicide note, warnings, violent methods, lethal poisons.

Prevention

Easy access to, and early and accurate diagnosis by, G.P. psychiatrist and voluntary agency are important. The Samaritans and other suicide agencies do useful work with potential suicides and parasuicides although there is no evidence that they reduce suicide rates. Prevention on a large scale must be directed to countering or minimising social isolation and to reducing alcohol consumption and abuse. All doctors have a duty to prescribe responsibly and to restrict access to drugs by avoiding large and repeated prescriptions. The public should be encouraged to clear out medicine cupboards regularly. Restrictions on barbiturates led in the 1970s to increased use of benzodiazepines (less dangerous in overdoses) and tricyclic antidepressants (more dangerous). The change to natural gas has been helpful: asphyxia is less lethal than carbon monoxide poisoning.

FURTHER READING

Alvarez A 1971 The savage god. Penguin, Harmondsworth
Greer S et al 1966 Aetiological factors in attempted suicide. British Medical Journal 2: 1352-1355
Maddison D, Mackey K H 1966 Suicide: the clinical problem. British Journal of Psychiatry 112: 693-703
Stengel E 1964 Suicide and attempted suicide. Penguin, Harmondsworth

17

Psychiatry and general practice

Psychiatrists see only the tip of an iceberg of patients. Psychiatric admissions and out-patient attendances may include the most severe and intractable cases and most of the functional psychoses, but careful research in general practice shows that only one in twenty psychiatric patients are referred to psychiatrists. In a typical practice psychological factors will be important in a third of patients seen; and 15 per cent of patients seen will have a mild, 3 per cent a moderate and 1.4 per cent a severe psychiatric disorder. It is only from these last two groups that referrals to psychiatrists are made.

The symptoms in these mild disorders are usually depressive. They occur largely in working class women in response to stressful life events, especially deaths, illness, unemployment, increasing financial difficulties and children in trouble. Those particularly vulnerable have three or more children under 14, no employment outside the home, lack a confiding relationship with anyone, especially a boyfriend or husband, and have lost a parent, usually the mother, before the age of 11 (Brown). Most of these reactions are short-lived and have a good prognosis.

Specialist referral

The family doctor has the difficult task of selection. Some patients select themselves, demanding a psychiatric opinion, others cannot be persuaded to risk the stigma of being labelled in this way.

Suicidal risk, or doubt about it, is high among the indications.

Acute psychosis, rare in any one practice, will usually require an urgent opinion or admission. The *perplexed adolescent* who may have schizophrenia, and those patients who show *intellectual impairment* require specialist investigation.

Uncommon conditions, like obsessional neurosis, are best seen by a specialist. The family doctor should know which patients are likely to benefit from behaviour therapy and more intensive psychotherapy than he can offer. He should never attempt to refer a patient to a psychiatrist without informing the patient, or try to have the specialist collude in pretending that he is someone else. Reassurance and explanation before referral can be helpful. Many patients still believe that psychiatric referral implies madness or that psychiatrists have no medical qualifications, and must be told that psychiatrists deal with many problems apart from psychosis.

Psychotropic prescribing

Psychotropic drugs make up over 17 per cent of all prescriptions, and cost the country many million pounds annually. The 'benzodiazepine bonanza' and the vast range of antidepressants available have raised patient expectations of a pill for all ills. It is difficult for the conscientious doctor to avoid giving a prescription to the anxious or mildly depressed patient when time is short and the patient demands it, although many patients would be better without it and helped more by discussion of their problems and reassurance. The bulk of benzodiazepines are used as expensive placebos. Although they may cause some dependence they are safer than barbiturates which cause severe problems of dependence. The risks of phenothiazines (jaundice, etc.) and antidepressants (cardiac arrhythmias, fits) should be borne in mind and they should only be prescribed thoughtfully. Any patients given a psychotropic drug may take an *overdose*. This should constantly be considered when choosing a drug and determining the quantity prescribed. Most doctors limit their prescribing to one or two drugs from each group, become familiar with them and resist the siren calls of new drug advertising until fully convinced about safety and efficacy. Repeat prescriptions must be regularly reviewed to avert abuse and dependence.

Psychotherapy

Time is the enemy of good psychiatry in general practice. Some practitioners dispute their responsibility for dealing with personal problems. Those interested set aside time for longer interviews with such patients and often find that the information and insight gained saves time in future management. The doctor learns when to reassure and when to explore further; how to reassure different types of patients, and how to use ventilation, exhortation, discussion and other brief psychotherapeutic techniques. Everyone develops a personal style, an essential part of the family doctor's efficacy. Some of this is developed unconsciously, based on the individual doctor's personality, but much can be learned by studying good examples.

In all practices a substantial minority of *chronic neurotic* patients accumulates. This population contains individuals with symptoms of chronic anxiety and depression, often with multiple handicaps, inadequate ineffectual personalities, low intelligence, and with backgrounds of social deprivation. They become dependent on the doctor, the practice resources, and on repeat prescriptions. Their efficient management is a continuing challenge. They may seem an ungrateful and unrewarding group, but are often kept functioning with the minimum of support and constant efforts to limit or diminish their dependence.

The family doctor as team leader

As well as working from time to time with the psychiatrist, who may do clinics in the health centre and make domiciliary visits, the family doctor as the leader of the primary care team must know what other agents or agencies may help his patient. Increasingly, psychiatric nurses are working in the community in *crisis intervention* teams, and following up and giving maintenance treatment to discharged patients. Social workers have an important role to play in psychiatric care and many have special psychiatric training and experience. Voluntary agencies should also be utilised: CRUSE, the organisation for widows, Alcoholics Anonymous and the Council for Alcoholism, Telephone Samaritans, and the Marriage Guidance Council. There are also several organisations for other specific groups of patients, e.g. phobics, schizophrenics.

18

Mental handicap

Mental handicap (amentia, oligophrenia) is a defect of intelligence existing from birth or from an early age. The English Mental Health Act, 1959, prefers 'mental subnormality' and recognises subnormality and severe subnormality. The Scottish Act of 1960 retains the older 'mental deficiency' and makes no subdivision. While low intelligence is essential, a low IQ is not the sole criterion. Personality and associated physical defects have significant effects on educability, and social competence has always been the main diagnostic criterion.

Prevalence
Two to three per cent of the population have some degree of mental handicap; they are gradually identified between birth and 14 years, after which the figure remains steady. Some 70 per cent live in the community. For every case of severe subnormality (IQ less than 30) there are 4 cases of moderate subnormality (IQ less than 50) and 15 mild cases of mild subnormality (IQ less than 75). Severe cases have a prevalence of 3.7/1000. Subnormality is nine times more common in social class 5 than in social class 1 and 2. It is higher in rural areas, and in males (1.3 to 1). There is a family history of subnormality in 17 per cent and of mental illness in 4 per cent.

Aetiology
There are two main types — organic and subcultural. The latter group comprises those individuals of low intelligence who can be expected to occur at one tail of the normal distribution curve. Intelligence is normally distributed in the population, and most intelligence tests are standardised with a mean IQ of 100 and a standard deviation of 15. The subnormal population is usually defined as having an IQ of more than two standard deviations below the mean, i.e. an IQ under 70. The rates quoted above for different degrees of defect illustrate the effects of the probability distribution and subcultural defect. In severe defect

— below IQ 50 — there are higher numbers than would be expected by chance (a 'bulge in the tail'), and the vast majority of this group have organic brain disease, compared with only 25 to 50 per cent in those with IQ's of 50 to 70.

Multiple handicap is common. A substantial minority has associated psychosis or neurosis, and up to 40 per cent show difficult behaviour in childhood.   Accompanying   handicaps   include   poor   physical development, sensory defects such as deafness and poor vision, cerebral palsy and epilepsy. Few with severe handicap can find employment, but above IQ 50 education, upbringing, social class and temperament, together with associated handicaps all play a part in the final achievement or failure.

Diagnosis and assessment

Antenatal

Amniocentesis: a developing area of early diagnosis, together with ultrasound, foetoscopy and foetal blood sampling. Tissue culture used to detect chromosomal abnormalities, enzyme defects and sex of the infant. May prove useful in older mothers with high risk of Down's syndrome, if an existing child has a genetic defect and risk is high, or if the disorder suspected is sex linked. Alphafoetoprotein estimation in amniotic fluid and blood now used to detect neural tube defects (spina-bifida): may also indicate foetal death. Risk of error: 1 in 1000.

Infancy

Always suspect subnormality when there has been anoxia and when there is low birth weight, dysplasia, cerebral palsy, convulsions or small cranial circumference. Probably 1 per cent of live births show serious retardation, but at 7 years only 0.4 per cent have IQ's below 50, the effect of *selective mortality*.

Investigations in suspected cases include chromosome studies, amino-acid chromatography, specific blood and urine tests for inborn errors of metabolism and detection of specific antibodies in mother and child. Developmental scales are available for diagnosis in infancy and childhood.

Childhood: many identified by failure to stand, walk or talk at the normal times.

School: milder degrees of subnormality are commonly diagnosed in the early school years through educational difficulties.

Classification

Organic causes

1. Prior to conception
   a. Chromosomal, e.g. Down's syndrome
   b. Genetic, single, e.g. inborn errors, or multifactorial
2. Pre-natal and peri-natal
   a. Maternal infections (rubella, toxoplasmosis, syphilis, cytomegalic inclusion body disease)
   b. Fetal infections (encephalopathies, maternal toxaemia)
   c. Maternal malnutrition — rare
   d. Perinatal damage (hypoxia, birth injury)
   e. Kernicterus
   f. Drugs or alcohol
   g. Exposure to radiation.

Down's syndrome (mongolism)

Described by John Langdon Down in 1866. Due to chromosomal abnormality. Various forms, but 95 per cent due to trisomy 21, an extra small acrocentric chromosome in group G, giving 47 rather than 46 chromosomes, Caused by non-disjunction during meiosis of the oöcyte, i.e. the ovum is involved and not the sperm. More common in older mothers; compared with a 25-year-old mother, a mother of 40 has 20 times the risk and a mother aged 45, 50 times the risk. Mongols born to young mothers usually show a different abnormality: translocation, in which there are 46 chromosomes, one of which is large and atypical. Clinically, mongolism is common: 1 in 700 live births, but up to 50 per cent die in the first year. Mongols formerly had a short life due to infection, but those who survive infancy now live longer. All show varying degrees of subnormality. In infancy hypotonia and hyperflexibility are found. There are multiple abnormalities: microcephaly, flat face, sloping eyes with epicanthic fold, big tongue and short neck; broad, flat hands with Simian crease and short fingers; congenital heart lesions, infertility, temperament jovial, often musical. In early pregnancy may now be identified by amniotic cell culture.

Metabolic abnormalities

Acquired
   a. Hypoglycaemia
   b. Hyperbilirubinaemia (kernicterus)
   c. Hypothyroidism (cretinism)
   d. Hypoproteinaemia

e. Hypercalcaemia
f. Lead poisoning
Inborn
a. Lipid
b. Carbohydrate
c. Amino acids.

Inborn errors of metabolism are interesting but very rare: acquired abnormalities are four times as common.

Acquired metabolic abnormality

Kernicterus: from Rh or ABO incompatibility or in prematurity. When level of unconjugated serum bilirubin exceeds 20 mg/100 ml, damage takes place in basal ganglia and cerebellum. Often hypertonus, cyanosis, convulsions with later choreo-athetosis, deafness and subnormality. Antenatal detection and exchange transfusion.

Hypothyroidism (Cretinism) has various causes: enzyme deficiencies, absent or maldeveloped thyroid, ingestion of drugs, e.g. phenylbutazone, PAS. Symptoms include: persistent jaundice, lethargy, protruding tongue and umbilical hernia; early thyroid treatment essential.

Inborn metabolic abnormality

All autosomal recessives. Rare — 1 in 10 000 to 1 in 50 000. Caused by deficient enzyme blocking a metabolic reaction: symptoms arise from accumulation of lipids, carbohydrate or amino acids before the block, or deficiency beyond the block.

Lipid disorders include Tay-Sachs' disease (ganglioside), Gaucher's disease (cerebroside) and Niemann-Pick disease (sphingomyelin). Commoner in Jews, begin early, have a rapid fatal course.

Connective tissue disorders (mucopoly-saccaroidoses) include Hurler's syndrome (gargoylism).

Carbohydrate disorders include galactosaemia, in which there is jaundice, cataracts, proteinuria and galactosuria. Treatable.

Amino acid disorders: best known is phenylketonuria. Infants are screened by Guthrie inhibition test on blood for raised phenylalanine levels. The defect is in transforming phenylalanine to tyrosine from a deficiency of the enzyme phenylalanine hydroxylase. Occurs 1 in 12 000 births. No physical abnormalities, but often have blue eyes, fair hair and dermatitis. May be fits. Treatment: Phenylalanine free diet, artificial and unpalatable, must be adhered to in childhood as long as child will tolerate it. Can be stopped in adult life, but resumed during pregnancy.

Neurological defects

Sturge-Weber syndrome: naevoid defect. Fits, hemiplegia, naevi (port wine stains) especially on face and neck. Venous angioma of pia; calcification of skull on X-ray. Hemispherectomy may help.

Tuberous sclerosis (epiloia). Sclerotic nodules in brain, epilepsy. Tumours elsewhere, especially kidneys and heart. Epilepsy. Skin lesions: adenoma sebaceum, fibromatosis, phakomata.

Laurence-Moon-Biedl Syndrome: mental defect, pigmentary degeneration of the retinae, obesity, hypogenitalism, polydactyly. Usually familial.

Bony defects

Genetic microcephaly: probably single recessive gene.

Hypertelorism: great breadth between eyes, due to abnormality of base of skull.

Oxycephaly: tower skull or steeple-head. Rarely associated with defect. Hypertelorism and oxycephaly need not be associated with subnormality.

Treatment and care

Patients should be cared for at home where possible but the stresses on other members of the family must be weighed. Boredom and overcrowding produce disturbed behaviour, and drugs (e.g. anticonvulsants) may further impair performance. Education is essential and should emphasise practical social skills — learning to wash, dress, eat, travel and work. Subnormals with an IQ of 50 or over can benefit from some form of schooling. Most defectives in the community are capable of some form of work and this may be in an occupation centre or sheltered workshop if open employment cannot be found. Very severely handicapped cases, cases with multiple handicaps or complicated by severe behaviour disorder (e.g. aggressiveness, disinhibited sexual behaviour) or psychotic illnesses will require care in hospital possibly throughout life. Prevention involves the paediatrician and obstetrician. Genetic counselling is developing in importance.

FURTHER READING

Forrest A D, Ritson B, Zealley A 1973 New perspectives in mental handicap. Churchill Livingstone, Edinburgh

19

Child and adolescent psychiatry

Aetiology
Genetic factors are important. Wide individual variations in mood, level of activity, attention span are found in infants, and sex differences in aggressive behaviour are evident at two years. These temperamental differences may modify parental response. Emotionally disturbed children have often been difficult babies. Personality differences noted at three years accurately predict adult personality. The child *is* father of the man.

For normal development, infants must form attachments and bonds (selective attachments persisting over a long period). *Separation* from parents, e.g. by hospital admission, is most stressful for children between six months and four years, but children can be trained to accept separations gradually. Short separations can lead to acute but brief distress. One long separation rarely does permanent emotional damage, but *repeated* hospitalisation in a child from an unhappy home often causes psychiatric problems.

Other damaging stresses on children include moving house, bereavement and a broken home. The latter is especially associated with conduct disorders. The associated *marital discord* is more important than the parents' separation. Children of one parent families have more psychiatric problems than average; children of working mothers do not.

Delinquency is associated with particular geographical areas which have poor neglected housing, overcrowding, low family income and high adult crime rates. Children in *inner cities* are twice as likely to have psychiatric disorder as those from elsewhere and to come from overcrowded, unhappy homes with disturbed parents. *Schools* with high rates of teacher and pupil turnover have more disturbed children. *Immigrant* children, especially West Indian, have high rates for conduct disorders.

Classification
A World Health Organisation Committee recommended that children be assessed on four dimensions: (1) clinical psychiatric syndrome; (2)

intelligence; (3) organic factors and (4) psychosocial factors. Clinically, children show the same range of psychiatric disorders as adults: psychoneurosis, psychosomatic disorders and psychosis. The vast majority can be divided into two groups:

1. With predominantly neurotic symptoms. These children suffer from anxiety, phobias, shyness, sleep and appetite disorders and tics. Most grow up to be stable adults.

2. With predominantly conduct disorders; stealing, aggression, lying, over-activity, truancy. Poor prognosis in adult life with much crime, alcoholism, psychiatric admission, poor work record.

Children with behaviour disorders are usually disturbed either at home or at school; only in severe cases at both. About 7 per cent of 10 to 11 year olds have some kind of psychiatric disorder. Boys have twice as much as girls and more often have conduct disorders.

A few disorders are specific to childhood and adolescence, e.g. early childhood *autism*, the *hyperkinetic syndrome* and *anorexia nervosa*. *Specific developmental disorders* include dyslexia, stammering, enuresis, encopresis and 'clumsy children'.

Specific syndromes

Nocturnal enuresis

Common in early years. At 14 years drops to 1 in 35. More frequent in males of below average intelligence living in poor social conditions. Strong family history. Five per cent urinary infections. May be neurotic, e.g. regression after birth of a younger sibling, or developmental. Treatment: conditioning by pad and bell (see p. 110), imipramine 25 or 50 mg at night in older children; prolonged treatment is necessary. *Encopresis:* Soiling; rarer than enuresis. Usually retention with overflow. Normal intelligence; may be neurotic or developmental. Treatment: unrewarding, but 50 per cent spontaneous recovery in two years, and all recover before adult life.

Stuttering

Two groups. First are dull, poor social background, often birth injury. The second, average or above average intelligence, ambitious families with worrying obsessional mothers. In both groups the anxiety engendered by stuttering may lead to secondary neurotic disorders. Speech therapy helpful.

Early childhood autism

A form of childhood psychosis beginning from birth or in the first three years. Not schizophrenia, which is rare and occurs later in childhood. Now generally agreed to be an organic condition —

formerly attributed to upbringing or the parents' personalities. The central defect is a difficulty in comprehension and the use of language. Rare — about 1 in 2000 school children. Three boys affected for every girl. Parents tend to be intelligent. Symptoms comprise lack of speech comprehension, mutism or abnormal speech, with echolalia, avoidance of the personal pronoun, monotonous mechanical voice. Difficulty in copying movements, flicking movements of hands, spinning and jumping movements. Paradoxical response to sounds. Resistance to change of routine. Socially aloof, live in a world of their own. Often tantrums. When testable, only 30 per cent have an IQ above 55. A third develop fits in adolescence or adult life. Differential diagnosis: deafness, partial blindness, elective mutism, mental subnormality. Prognosis: poor. Sixty per cent unchanged, only 15 per cent find open employment. Best with higher IQs.

School refusal ('school phobia')

Relatively rare. Peak age 11 to 12 years. Often precipitated by change of school or illness in parents, grandparents. Mostly boys, intelligence average. Well behaved children doing well at school, often anxious and shy. Increasing anxiety, often with abdominal pain and vomiting, culminating in refusal to go to school. Quite distinct from truancy. Mothers often over-protective, subject to depression. Most due to separation anxiety rather than fear of school. Treatment may necessitate admission, residential school or temporary separation from parents.

Tics (habit spasms)

Sudden, brief, often repeated movements involving a group of muscles. Have no purpose but usually based on purposive movements, e.g. blinking, head shaking, coughing. Most common is eye blinking; tics decline in frequency from head to feet. Found in 10 per cent aged 6 to 7 years. Twice as common in boys. Often family history of tics. Children average or above in intelligence, well behaved. Often associated with emotional disturbance; sometimes with speech disorders, obsessions and hypochondriasis.

The prognosis is good. Most are shortlived, the others spontaneously improve in adolescence. The very rare *Gilles de la Tourette syndrome* comprises multiple severe tics with compulsive swearing, and has a poor outlook.

Hyperkinetic syndrome

Overactive from an early age, sleeping little, wearing out clothes and shoes, unable to sit still. Dangerously impulsive. Distractable, short attention span, day dreaming and lack of perseverance. Excitable, frequent temper tantrums. Sometimes associated with organic brain disease, epilepsy or low IQ, but often not. Five times more common in boys, not a rare condition. Excess of minor neurological abnormalities — incoordination, clumsiness. Parents have above average rates for personality disorders and alcoholism. Children have similar risk in adult life. Prognosis is poor. Some respond to large doses of Ritalin (methyl phenidate) or to imipramine.

Elective mutism

Neurotic disorder in which child, usually male, is persistently mute in selected circumstances, e.g. at school. Most are solitary, over-dependent on parents. Treatment by change of environment or admission.

Adolescent psychiatry

The adolescent years are a time of major change for the individual. A *growth spurt* in early adolescence (13-14 for boys, 10-12 for girls) is followed soon after by *sexual maturation*. The adolescent has become physically different in a very short time and is faced with a strenuous *psychological adjustment* to these changes. Throughout adolescence intellectual maturation progresses. Although IQ does not continue to rise there is an increase in logical and abstract reasoning. Emotionally the adolescent strives for maturity and independence, particularly from his parents, but finds it difficult to give up the security and dependence of home and parents. His ambivalent feelings lead to frequent inconsistencies in behaviour. This 'in between' state is accompanied by mild feelings of depression and emptiness in 50 per cent of adolescents. Erikson described adolescence as a time of *identity crisis* when the individual has to decide who he is, what he can do and what he will make of his life. *Social* pressures are plentiful. He must learn many new roles at this time — changing from school to work, from child to parent. There is much pressure to conform to his peer group, whose standards differ sharply from those of parents. It should be emphasised that although minor conflicts are common, serious and persistent difficulties between adolescents and their parents are rare.

In a study of 14 year olds in the Isle of Wight, 20 per cent had evidence of psychiatric disorder, but half of these were not handicapped by their symptoms either at school or at home. A survey of urban teenagers showed that 6 per cent of boys and 3 per cent of girls had severe disorders. In general, rates for psychiatric disorder are higher than those for adults. Those who are disordered communicate poorly with their parents.

Types of adolescent disorder

As with children, adolescent disorders are best classified as behavioural (conduct) or emotional (neurotic). Many adolescents show both.

Neurotic disorder. As adolescence advances the symptoms approach those seen in adults. Depression and anxiety are common, the content of thought being the normal concerns of the age group magnified; appearance, sexual problems, status with friends are frequent preoccupations. School refusal in adolescence is a sign of severe neurotic difficulty.

Conduct disorder. More common in boys from disturbed families. Antisocial behaviour in a wide range of settings. Poor relations with others — not to be confused with delinquency. The number of delinquents showing psychiatric disorder is not much higher than average. Often associated with reading difficulties.

Anorexia nervosa

Common and increasing disorder of adolescent girls. Occurs in 1 in 150 girls in this age group. Only 1 in 20 patients are male. Begins with wish to diet and feeling fat. Progressive weight loss with early amenorrhoea, patient quickly becomes emaciated, but maintains she feels normal and looks normal. Claims to be eating adequately. Often self-induced vomiting and excessive purging: both in secret. May be intermittent over-eating (bulimia) especially after treatment. Patient very resistant to accepting treatment. Potentially serious. In those whom the condition lasts for ten years the later mortality may be 10 per cent. Often disturbed body image.

Weight falls in typical case to 30 to 35 kg. Best regarded as a phobic avoidance of adolescent weight gain and the physical and psychological changes of puberty. Treatment: target weight of at least 50 kg must be set and agreed. In-patient care usually essential with good nursing, high doses of phenothiazines and psychotherapy. Extended and careful follow-up.

Other problems

Suicide rare but rates rise in adolescence. Often taller than average and above average intelligence. *Attempted* suicide very common. May be associated with parental death.

Affective disorder is rare, *schizophrenia* more likely. Insidious onset cases may be difficult to distinguish from the normal difficulties of a shy adolescent with identity problems. *Brain damage* resulting from road traffic accidents is a growing problem. *Drug abuse* is common in adolescence and *alcoholism* increasing.

Treatment methods

In emotional disorders of childhood family relationships are often relevant and most child psychiatric clinics employ a treatment team including doctor, social worker, psychologist, nurse and play therapist. Individual or group therapy with the family members as well as the child is used. Residential treatment in hospital or special boarding school may be needed when the home is unsatisfactory or where the behaviour disorder cannot be contained by out-patient care alone. Drug treatments are less often used than with adults but tranquillisers and antidepressants are of value. ECT and psychosurgery are seldom, if ever, needed.

Treatment services

Many adolescents do not seek medical help with their symptoms. Some psychiatrists specialise in this age group, but many are seen by adult psychiatrists (e.g. self-poisonings, anorexia) while child psychiatrists often are involved with the younger adolescent, especially those with school difficulties. Interviewing and treating adolescents poses problems for the doctor who is usually seen as an agent of parental authority. The young doctor has an advantage in dealing with teenagers. Severely disturbed teenagers are best managed in a special adolescent unit with appropriate facilities — social and educational — rather than an adult hospital.

FURTHER READING

Baker P 1979 Basic child psychiatry. Staples Press, London
Rutter M 1975 Heoping troubled children. Penguin, Harmondsworth
Rutter M, Madge N 1976 Cycles of disadvantage: a review or research. Heinemann, London
Stone FH, Koupernik C 1978 Child psychiatry for students. Churchill Livingstone, Edinburgh
Valentine CL 1970 The normal child and some of his abnormalities. Penguin, Harmondsworth
Winnicott DW 1969 The child, the family and the outside world. Penguin, Harmondsworth

20

Forensic psychiatry

More than other doctors, the psychiatrist comes into contact with the law. Psychiatric patients, because of their disturbed behaviour, are likely to clash with society — hence the Mental Health Acts — and may encounter the police or the courts as a result. Forensic psychiatry is a growing subject, because there is growing interest in research, prevention, treatment and rehabilitation of the criminal rather than simple punishment. Not all criminals, of course, suffer from a psychiatric abnormality; one of the doctor's tasks is to distinguish those who do. This chapter gives a brief selection of psychiatrically important topics.

Crime
Crime is associated with youth and the male sex. There are 9 male offenders for every female and 33 male prisoners for every female. The largest increases in crime in the last 30 years have been in males between 14 and 21 years and the highest rates for theft and violent offences are in this age group. Studies of young male offenders show that they are of mesomorphic body build, extraverted, emotionally unstable, and condition poorly — they do not learn quickly from experience or punishment. They come from large families where there has been little parental control or from broken homes, are usually intellectually dull, of lower social class, and from areas of high crime.

Publicity gives a false impression of sex offences and crimes of violence which account for less than 5 per cent of all offences. About 2 per cent of all offenders are psychotic or mentally defective. Special hospitals for psychiatric patients who are potentially dangerous or criminal account for less than 1 per cent of psychiatric beds. There are more epileptics in the prison population than would be expected, but they are no more likely to commit violent crimes.

Violent criminals are of two types: under-controlled, habitually aggressive men with records of repeated minor violence (65 per cent have abnormal EEG's); over-controlled, older men who commit a single act of major violence, usually involving a relative (24 per cent have abnormal EEG's).

Murder

Rare. Psychiatric disorder in one-third. Associated with drinking (55 per cent in a Scottish series) and with subsequent suicide of the murderer (10 per cent in Scotland, up to 30 per cent in England). 25 per cent of the victims are strangers, 35 per cent close family relatives or lovers and the remainder acquaintances. 40 per cent of all women victims are killed by their husband. Matricide rare, usually by schizophrenics. Sexual murders very rare. Epileptics not more likely to commit murder.

Three syndromes are a major risk:

1. Sadistic murderers with interests in black magic, Nazi souvenirs, guns and bondage perversions.

2. *Morbid jealousy* (Othello syndrome). Accounts for 10 per cent of murders. The man develops a delusional belief in the infidelity of his wife. There is a five year history of a well developed paranoid delusional system, with complicated accusations and searches for non-existent evidence. The most dangerous syndrome in psychiatry.

3. Suicidal depression. The murderer believes that his wife and family would be happier dead and attempts to join them after the murder.

XYY syndrome

At the State Hospital Carstairs in 1965, 9 of 315 male patients were found to have abnormal sex chromosome complements, in the form of an extra Y chromosome — the XYY karyotype. The finding was confirmed in other institutions for psychiatric offenders, and shown to be associated with height (average 5ft 10in), below average intelligence, and a record of crime against property from an early age. The patients did not usually come from criminal families or cultures. The percentage is higher than in the general population but it is estimated that for every XYY identified there must be 100 'at large', and the significance of the findings remains uncertain.

Shoplifting

The main female crime. Only 6 per cent are professionals, 60 per cent are foreign born. Many are teenagers but there is a large group in the 45 to 55 group. In first offenders 20 per cent have psychiatric symptoms, in recidivists 30 per cent. One third have gynaecological symptoms, some menopausal but usually pre or post-natal or post-hysterectomy. In a 10 year follow-up 9 per cent required in-patient psychiatric treatment. The psychiatric symptoms are depressive. There is usually evidence of repressed resentment and ideas of self-punishment. In these cases the shoplifting is impulsive, articles of little value are taken, with little or no attempt at concealment. It is often provoked by a depressing event, but the woman frequently denies problems which are obvious to others, e.g. feelings of ageing, unwantedness and neglect by husband and children. Male shoplifters rare, usually take books. Juvenile shoplifting a group activity.

Prostitution

Prostitutes have a high incidence of mental abnormality. A study of a prison population showed that 25 per cent were alcoholic, 25 per cent were drug dependent, 25 per cent had a history of parasuicide, and 25 per cent had a variety of physical deformities and illnesses. Fifteen per cent were, or had been, psychiatrically ill, and 15 per cent were homosexual or bisexual.

Non-accidental injury to children

There are four main types of child damage: *Infanticide,* in which a mentally ill or defective mother kills her infant; *the wasted and neglected child,* the product of an inadequate mother and home; *deliberate sustained cruelty* by a sadistic parent; and *the battered baby syndrome,* increasingly reported in recent years.

'*Battered baby syndrome*'. The *child* is usually 3 years, there is a delay in reporting injury, denial of assault and a discrepancy between history and findings. There may be bruising, subdural haematoma, single or multiple fractures, ruptured liver and typical lacerations inside the mouth. Usually one particular child in the family is singled out, often the first or the last. One-third are illegitimate or unwanted. The *parents* are in their twenties, the mother of low intelligence, pregnant or premenstrual, the father unemployed and with a criminal record. The parents were sometimes ill-treated in their own childhood. They are superficially co-operative, the child is well dressed and well nourished, but there are marital and financial problems. Few are psychopathic or mentally ill.

Thorough investigation is necessary in suspected cases. The family doctor may not suspect the possibility of battering. The future safety of the children is paramount. If no-one intervenes there is a 60 per cent chance of further injury or death, and a 1 in 13 chance of a subsequent child being battered. Many agencies must be involved in care and follow-up on a team basis.

Battered wives

More than 1 in 500 marriages. 40 per cent men exposed to violence in childhood, 50 per cent wives lost a parent in childhood. Wives have better intelligence and work records than the husband. Alcoholism a major problem in husbands; 10 to 20 per cent of the wives drink heavily. May be morbid jealousy (see p. 97). May be a past history of incest or rape. Promiscuity common. Poor social conditions often, but occurs in all classes. Injuries often concealed or come to medical attention after some delay; mostly head and neck. Wives may be typed as inadequate, provocative or very competent. Treatment: social help offered to wife and children; open door and restricted admission hostels. Exclude or treat disorders in the husband: alcoholism, EEG abnormalities, atypical depression. Many cases are chronic, continuing for decades.

FURTHER READING

Gillies H 1976 Homicide in the West of Scotland. British Journal of Psychiatry 128: 105-127
Gunn J 1976 Sexual offenders. British Journal of Hospital Medicine 15: 57-65
Gunn J 1977 Criminal behaviour and mental disorder. British Journal of Psychiatry 130: 317-329
Patrick J A 1973 A Glasgow gang observed. Methuen, London
Pizzey E 1974 Scream quietly or the neighbours will hear. Penguin, Harmondsworth
Smith S M et al 1974 Social aspects of the battered baby syndrome. British Journal of Psychiatry 125: 568-582

21

Legal aspects of psychiatry

In contrast with other forms of illness, admission of all psychiatric patients to mental hospitals was in the past governed by legal procedures laid down in the *Lunacy and Mental Deficiency Acts.*

The Mental Health Acts (England 1959, Scotland 1960) provide for the care and treatment of mentally disordered persons, for their protection and for safeguarding their property and affairs. They ensure that wherever possible the mentally disordered patient can have the same ready access, without formality, to care and treatment as the patient suffering from a physical disorder. These Acts have been criticised for not providing sufficient protection for patients' civil rights and are being reviewed. New legislation may be made in 1981.

The Mental Health Act 1959

According to the Act, *mental disorder,* for which compulsory admission is permissible, means *mental illness* or *severe subnormality* at any age, a *psychopathic disorder* or *subnormality* in those under 21. Compulsory admission may be under various sections:

(*Section 25*). This is for observation over a period of 28 days. Application is made by the nearest relative or by a social worker (Mental Welfare Officer) and supported by two medical recommendations — one by a doctor with some knowledge of the patient, usually the G.P., and the other by a doctor approved by the Health Authority as having experience in psychiatry.

(*Section 29*). Secures admission for 72 hours. Only one doctor need make the application.

(*Section 26*). Permits compulsory treatment for up to one year. Patient has a right to appeal to a Mental Health Tribunal.

(*Section 60*). An order made by a court for the compulsory treatment of a patient convicted of a criminal offence.

(*Section 65*). Empowers superior courts to restrict the discharge of a patient. Home Office permission is then required for the patient to leave hospital.

(*Section 136*). Allows a police officer to take a mentally disordered person from a public place to hospital for 72 hours.

The Mental Health (Scotland) Act, 1960

Mental disorder is used as a general term to cover *mental illness* and *mental deficiency,* however manifested or caused. These are the only categories of mental disorder referred to in the Act.

Particular hospitals are no longer designated as mental hospitals or mental deficiency institutions. Special provision is made for 'State Hospitals' for patients with dangerous, violent or criminal propensities who require treatment under conditions of special security.

Provision of mental health services by local authorities

Local authorities are empowered to:

1. Provide residential accommodation
2. Exercise functions in respect of persons under guardianship, and supervise mental defectives
3. Ascertain mental deficiency in persons not of school age
4. Appoint Mental Health Officers (M.H.O.) to carry out duties relating to compulsory detention and guardianship
5. Provide ancillary and supplementary services.

The local authority must also arrange suitable training for mental defectives not already provided for by special schools.

Admission to hospital

It is specifically stated that nothing in the Act is to prevent a patient requiring treatment for mental disorder from being admitted to any hospital or nursing home and receiving treatment without formality, in the same way as patients are admitted to hospital for treatment for physical conditions.

Compulsory admission

(*Section 24*). Where the patient is unwilling to enter hospital the Act provides for:

1. Admission on the application of the nearest relative or a M.H.O., the recommendation of two doctors, and the approval of a Sheriff prior to admission
2. Subsequent periodic review of the need for detention
3. Right of appeal to the Sheriff against detention by patient or nearest relative
4. An independent central authority, the Mental Welfare Commission, with a right to visit patients, discharge a patient at any

time and to hear and investigate any complaint of wrongful or improper treatment.

The two medical practitioners must examine the patient separately. One must have special experience in the diagnosis or treatment of mental disorder and the other, where possible, should be the patient's general practitioner. Only one of the doctors may be on the staff of the hospital to which the patient is to be admitted and neither if the patient is to be treated privately.

The medical recommendations state:

1. The form of the patient's mental disorder (i.e. mental illness or mental deficiency)

2. That it is of a nature or degree warranting detention in hospital for treatment

3. That the interests of the patient's health and safety or the protection of other persons cannot otherwise be secured.

The Sheriff must approve the application and medical recommendations and may make his own enquiries. It the nearest relative objects he must be given a hearing in private. The completed Section 24 Order then permits detention in hospital for 28 days.

Emergency admission (Section 31). A patient may be removed to hospital on the strength of one medical recommendation in cases of urgency and detained for up to seven days. The recommendation must state that mental illness exists and where possible that consent of a relative has been obtained. The hospital which agrees to accept the patient usually arranges transport and escorts. During the seven day period the Section 24 Order should be completed.

Two classes of patient are not liable to compulsory admission if over 21:

1. Mental defectives who are able to lead an independent life and guard themselves against serious exploitation

2. Mentally ill persons with a persistent disorder manifested only by abnormally aggressive or seriously irresponsible conduct.

Patients in these classes already detained are to be reviewed with a view to discharge on reaching the age of 25.

Part V of the Act deals with patients concerned in criminal proceedings. The provisions of this part of the Act are now incorporated in the Criminal Procedure (Scotland) Act 1975. Courts may remand offenders to hospital for a psychiatric report. After trial the Court may make an Order for treatment. In certain circumstances a restriction may be placed on a patient's discharge from hospital. A patient who is 'insane and unfit to plead' will automatically receive a treatment order.

The Mental Welfare Commission is a statutory body set up by the Scottish Act to exercise a protective function for persons with mental disorder: it can investigate complaints by patients or their relatives about their treatment and can order a patient's discharge.

Legal considerations
Care and treatment of the psychiatric patient may involve a number of other legal considerations. For example:

Marriage and divorce
Formerly, husband or wife could obtain divorce on grounds of incurable insanity of the partner. Partner must have been continuously under care and treatment for mental illness for five years. Recent legislation in both Scotland and England makes divorce possible in a shorter time after irreconcilable breakdown of marriage and has superceded these provisions.

Marriage can be annulled if one of the parties at the time of the marriage was not able to understand the marriage contract or unable to manage his affairs. The patient, having recovered, can bring an action of nullity. Conversely, a petition for nullity will be upheld if the petitioner was unaware of the partner's insanity at the time of marriage, provided less than one year has elapsed since marriage.

Sterilisation and abortion
In Britain sterilisation and therapeutic termination of pregnancy may be carried out legally for medical reasons; the procedure and indications for termination are now regulated by the Abortion Act, 1967. The grounds recognised by the Act include risk to the life of the pregnant woman, risk of injury to the physical or mental health of the pregnant woman, risk of injury to the physical or mental health of the existing children of the family and substantial risk of physical or mental abnormality or serious handicap in the unborn child. The indications are broad and their interpretation in practice has not yet been established. The abortion is carried out with the permission of the patient on the recommendation of two doctors and has to be notified to the Chief Medical Officer of the Department of Health.

Criminal responsibility
The psychiatric state of the offender is given consideration in all types of legal proceeding. If minor offences occur in a person under psychiatric care he is seldom prosecuted. Attempted suicide is not a legal offence. It is common for an offender to be remanded for a medical report or to be placed on probation on the undertaking that he will accept medical treatment.

In more serious offences the accused may be found insane and unfit to plead and may be detained in a Special or State Hospital.

Diminished responsibility

Lesser degrees of psychiatric abnormality than insanity are taken into account where mental responsibility is impaired, e.g. by low intelligence or psychopathic personality, and in cases of homicide only, the charge may be reduced from murder to manslaughter by this defence.

Neurotic illness

A diagnosis of psychoneurosis may be considered in mitigation of sentence in minor offences but here legal responsibility is not diminished.

Property of mentally disordered persons

Where patients with mental disorder are unable to manage their affairs the Court of Protection arranges for this to be done. Such patients are supervised by the Lord Chancellor's Visitors.

In Scotland the law provides for the appointment of a *curator bonis* to manage the patient's affairs and the local authority has a duty to arrange for such an appointment if no other person has done so. The Mental Welfare Commission supervise patients who have a curator.

Testamentary capacity

A patient's mental disorder may make him unable to understand the implications of making a will. In these circumstances a court may make arrangements for the disposal of the patient's estate after his death.

FURTHER READING

BMA 1980 The handbook of medical ethics
Venables H D 1975 A guide to the law affecting mental patients. Butterworths, London

22

Psychological treatments

Psychotherapy

Psychotherapy may be broadly defined as any treatment designed to influence behaviour by verbal or non-verbal means, and includes techniques as varied as confession, reassurance, hypnosis, psychoanalysis and brain-washing. There is ample evidence from outside medicine that what one person says to another may greatly influence behaviour, and doctors have always realised the therapeutic, as well as the diagnostic value of intelligent history-taking. Historically much treatment relied on suggestion, reassurance and the doctor's prestige, administered directly or through placebo therapy. The doctor-patient relationship remains immeasurably important in all specialties.

Such psychotherapy is informal, unplanned, and usually lacks any theoretical foundation. Formal psychotherapy proceeds in a planned way and is based on a theory explaining the psychogenesis of the patient's complaints and the relationship between doctor and patient.

Freud and psychoanalysis

All modern psychotherapy owes much to Sigmund Freud (1856-1939), the originator of the theory and technique of psychoanalysis. His work has been criticised as unscientific, but his ideas permeate twentieth century thought and have perhaps been more influential outside medicine than within.

The theory of psychoanalysis includes:

1. The role of *unconscious* factors in normal and neurotic behaviour; known long before Freud and easily proven in experimental hypnosis. Freud developed the idea of an active or *dynamic unconscious*.

2. *Psychological determinism.* The view that seemingly chance or absurd dreams, slips of the tongue and neurotic symptoms have a meaning, usually unconscious and *symbolic*.

3. *Infantile sexuality.* Freud's *libido theory:* energy attached to the sexual instincts can be linked to different objects at different developmental stages. The oral phase lasts from birth to 18 months,

the anal stage from 18 months to 3 years and the phallic stage until seven, when there is a latency period until puberty. During the phallic stage boys develop the *Oedipus complex* in which the father is seen as a rival for mother's affection.

4. *Topographical model.* Freud's structural model of the mind comprising the id (instinctual, childlike, unconscious forces) the ego (conscious, rational, adult) and the superego (conscience, parental ideas).

5. *Psychogenesis.* The view that symptoms have psychological origins, particularly through conflict and anxiety and in childhood experiences.

6. *Mechanisms of defence.* Mental mechanisms that are often typical of the individual or a particular neurosis and are used to deal with anxiety. They include:

Projection: attributing ones own intentions (usually unconscious) to others, e.g. in paranoid personalities.

Reaction-formation: behaving consciously in a way opposite to unconscious wishes, e.g. the over-polite person concealing hostility.

Rationalisation: attempting to provide logical reasons for emotional and illogical attitudes.

Displacement: an undesirable idea is not allowed to reach consciousness but is transferred to a more acceptable object or person, e.g. an outburst of anger is directed at the cat instead of the parent.

Identification: modelling behaviour on that of another, e.g. the boy identifying with his father.

In developing the *technique* of psychoanalysis Freud used:

1. *Free association.* The patient is encouraged to say whatever enters his head at any time during the daily hour of treatment (the 'basic rule').

2. *Interpretation.* The analyst remains largely silent, refusing to ask or answer questions, but may offer interpretations of the patient's dreams, fantasies and behaviour.

3. *Analysis of the transference.* Transference phenomena are the feelings, positive and negative, developed by the patient for the doctor (the doctor may have *counter-transference* feelings). They have no realistic foundation in the present and are related to the patient's feelings for significant figures, usually parental, in the past, e.g. the patient may treat the male psychotherapist as though he were his father. Psychoanalysis, and indeed any kind of intensive psychotherapy, makes use of these feelings. Intellectual understanding of the patient's problems is insufficient and emotional understanding, as relived in transference, is essential for improvement.

4. *'Working through'*. Insight gained in the above way must be put into practical use in real life as part of successful treatment.

As a practical procedure, psychoanalysis occupies some five daily hours each week over several years and is carried out by a psychoanalyst, usually medically qualified, who himself has undertaken a lengthy training analysis. There are few analysts in the National Health Service and clearly they can treat only a handful of patients.

Freud had and has many disciples, some of whom, notably Adler and Jung, broke with the master and formed their own schools. C. G. Jung (1875-1961) did not agree with Freud's views on infantile sexuality, coined the terms 'introversion' and 'extraversion', and took a mystical view of a collective unconscious. Alfred Adler (1870-1937) paid more attention to the individual's willpower and to social factors. There have been many influential *Neo-Freudians*. In the U.S. Erich Fromm, H. S. Sullivan and K. Horney, and in Great Britain Anna Freud, Melanie Klein and R. Fairbairn have all added to psychoanalytic theory. Despite the multiplicity of theories and schools, studies of psychotherapists show that their actual practice differs surprisingly little. Current practice tends to more active participation by the therapist, concentration on interpersonal events in the present rather than the past, and on analysis of transference and the patient's typical defence mechanisms rather than to a search for traumatic events in the patient's childhood. Successful therapists have qualities of 'accurate empathy, non-possessive warmth, and genuineness'.

Indications for psychotherapy

Psychoneurosis and some personality and psychosomatic disorders. For intensive psychotherapy the patients selected are usually young, intelligent, highly-motivated, with an ability to verbalise freely and capacity for insight. Brief and supportive psychotherapy is used in all the milder psychiatric disorders.

Types of psychotherapy

Psychiatrists, and many others, practise psychotherapy of varying degrees of intensity, ranging from brief and infrequent interviews to weekly sessions of one hour continuing over months and years.

1. *Brief therapy*. A variety of techniques are exploited, usually in combination:

Ventilation, in which the patient confides, confesses, and is given the opportunity to ventilate his past and present difficulties.

Clarification, where problems are discussed and their nature and relations made clear.

Abreaction, verbalising emotionally charged material, with the release of anxiety, anger or grief.

Desensitisation, in which repetitive ventilation of feelings, as in mourning, has a therapeutic effect.

Suppression. The therapist acts in a directive and authoritarian way, using direct advice, orders, exhortation, persuasion and suggestion. Suggestibility may be increased by hypnosis or reinforced by drugs or placebos.

2. *Intensive psychotherapy.* Such treatment is usually practised by those with specialist training and includes psychoanalysis. In contrast to brief therapy the interviews are longer and more frequent. The therapist assumes a more neutral attitude, there is more detailed examination of the patient's past and present problems, and some analysis of the transference is used in the treatment.

3. *Group therapy.* Treating psychoneurotic patients in small groups, usually of 6 to 8 people, is more economical than individual psychotherapy and has advantages for patients with marked social and interpersonal difficulties. Defence mechanisms and transference reactions are seen, akin to those that occur in individual therapy, and are made use of by the therapist. Sessions are held weekly, last one to one and a half hours, and continue for one to two years. Group theory — about the type of leadership, the life of a group, interaction, etc. — uses social psychology and sociology as well as psychoanalysis as sources.

Group therapy has flourished in the social climate of the United States with a bewildering variety of techniques, much subject to fashion. *Psychodrama* was an early technique in which patients are encouraged to act out their problems and family conflicts by role-playing and improvisation. *'T' (training) groups* (Lewin) were developed as an educational group experience emphasising the present and self-disclosure. *Encounter* groups were developed to heighten awareness in normal people rather than patients and also emphasise group confession. *Transactional analysis* (Berne) which analyses the 'games people play', is another U.S. movement which has had wide success. There are many fringe groups with untrained leaders or run as self-help groups. They may attract potential patients, including the psychotic, and have a detrimental effect on them.

4. *Conjoint family therapy.* A form of psychotherapy in which one or two therapists see several members of a family together. It can be regarded as a special form of group therapy. As well as using analytic ideas it has made use of sociological concepts of role and of general

systems theory in explaining what happens in normal and pathological family relationships, e.g. scapegoating, when one member of the family is consistently blamed for all the family's problems. Unproven efficacy.

5. *Administrative therapy*. Because interpersonal relationships are so important in the genesis and treatment of psychiatric disorders, considerable attention is given nowadays to staff-patient relations in psychiatric hospitals and wards. The concept of the hospital as a *therapeutic community*, developed by Maxwell Jones, involves organising the hospital in a democratic way, with patients having a say in the conduct of their affairs, and staff relinquishing authoritarian habits. There must be free communications between doctors, nurses, other staff and patients, and all should feel able and have the opportunity to express their feelings to one another. To this end staff and patients meet regularly, and ward meetings become an extension of group psychotherapy. When such principles were neglected, patients became apathetic and experienced a loss of individuality, a condition which has been called *institutional neurosis*.

Effectiveness of psychotherapy

Despite its use over 80 years there are no entirely satisfactory trials of psychotherapy because of the technical difficulties of such research; those that have been completed are equivocal about the efficacy of psychotherapy. A well-known research project by Sloane (1975) compared three groups of patients, assigning them to 14 weekly analytic psychotherapy sessions, to a similar period of behaviour therapy, or to a waiting list. All patients improved including those on the waiting list who had had an initial assessment, telephone contact and emergency services as needed. The two groups having active treatment improved more than the 'control' group. There was little change in those results one and two years later.

Behaviour therapy

Behaviour therapy is the most active area of growth in psychotherapy. It has been developed largely by psychologists from their studies on experimental learning in man and animals. It attempts to change symptoms directly rather than seek for underlying causes, and assumes that neurotic symptoms stem from faulty learning. Many of its ideas are commonsensical and have long been used by parents and teachers.

Learning

The term is used to describe any relatively permanent change in behaviour resulting from past experience; it need not be intentional, nor need the learner be aware that he is learning.

Classical conditioning. First described by Pavlov (1849-1936). An unconditioned response (a dog salivating) to an unconditioned stimulus (sight or smell of food) is modified by pairing a conditioned stimulus (a bell ringing) with the unconditioned stimulus. After a number of trials the conditioned stimulus (bell) alone will produce the conditioned response (salivation). After a while *extinction* of the response will occur. The response can be *generalised* to other sounds or *discrimination* may be taught (e.g. high pitched bells).

Operant conditioning or instrumental learning involves changing the frequency with which a certain behaviour occurs in a particular situation. The typical experiment involves a pigeon in a Skinner box. When a lever is pecked, at first by accident, food enters the box. The pigeon learns to press the lever more frequently for the reward. The behaviour is *reinforced* by the reward — this can be done continuously, intermittently or at second hand. As well as *reward* training, animals can be trained to *escape* from or *avoid* painful stimuli. Operant learning can be complex, developed by successive approximations (*shaping*) and building up sequences (*chaining*). Avoidance responses are very lasting (e.g. agoraphobia). Mowrer's 2-factor theory explains this by:

1. development of a conditioned response pairing fear and the place to be avoided.

2. reinforcement of the avoidance. Fear occurs on approaching the place again and stops with avoidance.

Observational learning is found in human beings, e.g. *modelling* actions of others in sports and new social situations. It can teach others to do things and to avoid things.

Types of behaviour therapy

Systematic desensitisation. The first technique, developed by a South African psychiatrist, Wolpe (1969) from animal experiments on the principle of *reciprocal inhibition* of neurotic responses. If a response incompatible with anxiety can be made to occur at the same time as an anxiety provoking stimulus then the anxiety will be reduced. The patient's detailed history is used to construct a *hierarchy of responses* — from the least to the most anxiety provoking. He is taught relaxation exercises or relaxed by drugs and asked to imagine himself in the anxiety provoking situations — progressive desensitisation occurs.

Token economy. Severely socially handicapped patients in longstay wards may be remotivated by the use of tokens. The basic essentials of nursing care are provided, but extra food, attention, privileges are bought with tokens. The tokens are used by the staff as an operant conditioning device. The desired behaviour when it appears is immediately rewarded and shaped by tokens.

Aversion treatment. Pleasant but undesirable behaviour (alcoholism, deviant sexual fantasies) can be reduced by aversive conditioning, pairing the pleasant stimulus with an unpleasant response (alcohol and apomorphine, fantasy and electric shock). *Thought-stopping* techniques are used to abolish obsessional ruminations. The patient signals when they begin and the therapist shouts 'stop' or gives a shock to the patient. Later the patient may control the symptom by saying 'stop' to himself, or flicking a rubber band on the wrist to produce a painful stimulus.

Flooding and response prevention. Research on systematic desensitisation suggests that exposure to the feared object is the sole essential ingredient. *Flooding* involves direct prolonged contact with the feared object with the therapist's support, encouragement and modelling. In the treatment of obsessional rituals *response prevention* is a similar and effective treatment. Both require skilled therapists (often specially trained nurses) and may be very time consuming.

Social skills training. Argyle's work on social interaction led him to compare social skills to complex motor skills, capable of being broken down into separate parts and of being analysed in terms of cues, responses and feedback. Individuals with social difficulties can be taught social skills, often in groups. They can be *instructed* in how to move and what to say. They may *model* their performance from a live person or a TV film, *rehearse* the skill, be *socially reinforced* by the group's or therapist's compliments, and be given *feedback*, e.g. by watching a videotape, of their performance.

Other behavioural techniques. An animal model of neurosis is provided by Pavlov's dogs conditioned to a painful stimulus they cannot avoid. Subsequently put in an operant conditioning experiment where they can evade punishment they do not do so. Seligman has called this *learned helplessness* and compared it to the behaviour of people with neurotic depression. Treatment by *assertive training* may be helpful in such cases. A behavioural approach to *marital therapy* involves teaching the couple to *mutually reinforce* each other. Weekly contracts are made, in which each lists positive actions he would like the other to do. This 'giving to get' approach is also used in treating sexual dysfunction (see p. 66).

Biofeedback. The development of small, lightweight and sensitive electronic apparatus makes it possible for the patient to be given immediate, portable feedback on physiological activities not normally available to his conscious mind, e.g. pulse, EEG, alpha activity, psychogalvanic response (PGR), blood pressure, muscle activity. Much clinical experimentation is exploring the possibility that patients may thus be able to control responses normally not in awareness. Relaxation can certainly be facilitated and there have been suggestive results in tension headaches, migraine (temporal artery flow) and hypertension.

FURTHER READING

Argyle M 1974 Psychology of interpersonal behaviour. Penguin, Harmondsworth
Bloch S 1979 An introduction to the psychotherapies. OUP, Oxford
Brown D, Pedder J 1979 Introduction to psychotherapy. Tavistock, London
Eysenck H J 1975 Psychological theories and behaviour therapy. Psychological Medicine 5: 219-221
Jones E 1953 Life and work of Sigmund Freud. Penguin, Harmondsworth
Kovel J 1978 A complete guide to therapy. Penguin, Harmondsworth
Rogers C 1973 Encounter groups. Penguin, Harmondsworth
Sloane R B et al 1975 Short-term analytically oriented psychotherapy versus behaviour therapy. American Journal of Psychiatry 132: 373-377
Stafford-Clark D 1965 What Freud really said. Penguin, Harmondsworth

23

Drug treatment

Psychopharmacology

The development and asessment of new drugs in psychiatry pose special problems. Animal responses can provide only a rough comparison with possible effects on psychiatric symptoms, but many useful techniques exist. Motor behaviour, learning and memory, appetite and sexual activity can all be measured. Aggression in animals resembles irritability in man, and experimental neurosis (Pavlov) simulates fear and anxiety. As in some humans, the administration of reserpine to animals produces a state resembling retarded depression, which has been widely used to test the effects of new anti-depressants. The known effects of established psychotropic drugs on animals are utilised in screening new drugs.

In man, objective measures and rating scales are used when testing new drugs. Difficulties arise from the fluctuating course of many illnesses, and from lack of diagnostic precision, e.g. is a new drug for schizophrenia effective for all symptoms, in acute and chronic, hebephrenic and paranoid forms, etc.? The most serious obstacle of all is the *placebo reaction* arising from a number of non-specific factors, which may influence the patient's response:

a. *Patient factors:* sex, age, symptoms, personality

b. *Doctor factors:* the doctor's enthusiasm or lack of it has been shown to affect trial results

c. *Environment:* hospital or home, presence of other patients on the same drug

d. *Drug factors:* colour, taste, preparation (tablet, liquid, etc.), frequency, route — injections have more impact than oral medication.

Some degree of placebo response can be found in two-thirds of patients (and healthy people) and is not confined to patients with neurosis or personality disorders.

No new drug becomes established today without adequate controlled trial ('double-blind') against a placebo or the established remedy. Side effects, toxic effects and the risk of dependency must also be measured.

1. Drug treatments

Tranquillisers
  a. *Phenothiazines*

Examples:

Chlorpromazine hydrochloride (Largactil)

Indications:	Controls agitation and excitement and is used in the treatment of schizophrenia, agitated depression, manic states, drug and alcohol withdrawal and delirium.
Dosage:	75–1000 mg daily. Available as tablets of 10, 25, 50 and 100 mg. Also 25 mg/ml solution for injection. Average dose 300 mg daily.
Side effects:	Tachycardia, postural hypotension, dry mouth, constipation, drowsiness, skin rashes and increased sensitivity to sunlight. Parkinsonism with large doses. After two years or more of continuous treatment, rhythmic spontaneous movements appear especially around the mouth and in the tongue (*tardive dyskinesia*). May respond to tetrabenazine (Nitoman), 75–200mg daily, but usually irreversible. Phenothiazine dosage should be as low as possible and 'drug holidays' given during long term administration.
Toxic effects:	Impairment of liver function in 5–10 per cent of patients and more with high doses. Cholestatic jaundice in about 1 per cent. Agranulocytosis occurs rarely.

Trifluoperazine (Stelazine)

Indications:	As for chlorpromazine. More potent but less sedative effect. Available as 1 mg and 5 mg tablets, and 2, 10 and 15 mg 'spansules'. Average dose in schizophrenia 5 mg thrice daily.
Side effects:	In doses over 15 mg daily extrapyramidal symptoms are common: Parkinsonism, dyskinesias, muscle spasm. Initial restless phase (akathisia) common.

Fluphenazine hydrochloride (Moditen, Modecate)

Indications:	As for chlorpromazine. Slow release preparations fluphenazine enanthate (Moditen Enanthate) and fluphenazine decanoate (Modecate) 25 mg per ml given every 2–4 weeks are now widely used for maintenance treatment of schizophrenics — especially on an out-patient or day-patient basis.
Side effects:	Extra-pyramidal symptoms are common with the slow release forms and an anti-Parkinson drug e.g. orphenadrine (Disipal) 50–150 mg daily may be needed in addition.

Thioridazine hydrochloride (Melleril)

Indications:	As for chlorpromazine.
Dosage:	Up to 600 mg daily.
Side effects:	May be less frequent than with other phenothiazines.

Many other phenothiazine derivatives are on the market. These have no marked advantage over the examples mentioned above.

    Promazine (Sparine)
    Methotrimeprazine (Veractil)
    Prochlorperazine (Stemetil)
    Perphenazine (Fentazin)
    Pericyazine (Neulactil)
    Thiopropazate (Dartalan).

b. *Benzodiazepines*
Example:
Chlordiazepoxide (Librium)

Indications:	Anxiety and tension. Night sedation.
Dosage:	10–20 mg t.i.d.
Side effects:	Dizziness, nausea, irritability and disinhibited behaviour seen occasionally. Some recent evidence of drug dependence.

Other members of this group include:

Oxazepam (Serenid) 10–30 mg t.i.d.
Diazepam (Valium) 2–10 mg t.i.d.
Medazepam (Nobrium) 5–10 mg t.i.d.
Nitrazepam (Mogadon) 5–10 mg at night.
Lorazepam (Ativan) 1–2.5 mg t.i.d.
Flurazepam (Dalmane) 15–30 mg at night.
Clonazepam (Rivotril) 4–8 mg a day for epilepsy.
Chlorazepate (Tranxene) 15 mg at night.
Temazepam (Normison) 10–30 mg at night.
Clobazam (Frisium) 10 mg t.i.d.

c. *Miscellaneous group.* Many other tranquillising drugs are available and widely used. It is preferable to become familiar with the side effects and dosage of a few than to change too frequently.

Some popular members of the group are:

Chlormethiazole (Heminevrin) 0.5–1.0 G t.i.d. Often used for delirium and in the elderly. Some risk of dependence.
Haloperidol (Serenace) 0.5–5 mg t.i.d. Useful in acute mania. Doses of up to 80 mg a day have been used but with no consistent benefit.
Trifluoperidol (Triperidol) 0.5–2 mg t.i.d.
Flupenthixol (Depixol) 20–40 mg i.m. every 2 to 4 weeks. Used in chronic schizophrenia.
Pimozide (Orap) 2–8 mg daily. Used in schizophrenia. Advantage of single daily dose.
Fluspiriline (Redeptin) 2–20 mg i.m. every 1 to 2 weeks in schizophrenia.

Antidepressants
a. 'Tricyclic' group
Examples:
Imipramine hydrochloride (Tofranil)

Pharmacology:	An imino-dibenzyl derivative. It has both anti-cholinergic and adrenergic effects. It has no euphoriant effect when given to normal subjects. Its exact mode of action is unknown but it raises the levels of serotonin and catecholamines in the brain and produces EEG changes in the diencephalon where these substances are in their highest concentration. Other experimental evidence suggests that catecholamines play an important role in mood regulation.
Indications:	Imipramine can in most cases replace ECT. It is effective in endogenous depression, but less often helps reactive depressions. Retarded patients respond better than those who are agitated. Patients respond gradually in from one to four weeks, which is a disadvantage in potentially suicidal cases. Over 50 per cent of the endogenous depressions remit but relapse occurs if a maintenance dose is not given.
Dosage:	25–75 mg t.i.d.

Side effects: Dry mouth and difficulty in focusing (anti-cholinergic), attacks of sweating and flushing (adrenergic) are all common. Less commonly and with doses over 200 mg daily, tremors, muscle twitchings, dysuria and epilepsy (1-2 per cent). Headaches, insomnia and slight hypotension may occur. Some patients may become hypomanic during treatment. Cardiotoxic effects also found. In hypertensive patients on adrenergic blocking drugs may interfere with blood pressure control.

Amitriptyline hydrochloride (Tryptizol)

Pharmacology: Similar to imipramine but has some phenothiazine-like sedative action.
Indications: As for imipramine, useful for agitated depression.
Dosage: 25-75 mg t.i.d. 25-100 mg spansules at night.
Side effects: As for imipramine.

Others

Opipramol (Insidon), trimipramine (Surmontil), desipramine (Pertofan), nortriptyline (Aventyl, Allegron), dibenzepin (Noveril), doxepin (Sinequan), iprindole (Prondol), clomipramine (Anafranil), protriptyline (Concordin), dothiepin (Prothiaden).

b. *Miscellaneous group.* A number of related drugs similar in effect to the tricyclic group have been developed. For example:

Maprotiline (Ludiomil) 75-150 mg daily.
Mianserin (Bolvidon, Norval) 30-60 mg daily.
Viloxazine (Vivalan) 150-300 mg daily.
Nomifensine (Merital) 75-150 mg daily.
Flupenthixol (Fluanxol) 0.5-3 mg daily.
The indications for these drugs and their relative merits are still being assessed. Some are more expensive than the tri-cyclics described earlier.

c. *Monoamine-oxidase inhibitors (MAOIs)*

Example:

Phenelzine (Nardil)

Pharmacology: A hydrazine derivative. The action in depression is probably due to the ability to inhibit amine-oxidase. The function of the enzyme monoamine-oxidase is the breakdown of serotonin and catecholamines in the brain. Amine-oxidase inhibitors consequently raise the brain levels of serotonin and catecholamines.
Indications: Atypical or milder depressions, especially with evening worsening and phobias.
Dosage: 15-30 mg t.i.d.
Side effects: Dizziness, hypotension, hepatitis, urinary retention, insomnia. Severe headache with hypertension may occur, often after eating cheese and other substances rich in tyramine due to the inhibition of amine-oxidase and the pressor effects of the tyramine.
Precautions: Patients on this group of drugs must avoid cheese, meat extracts, peas and beans, yeast extracts, pickled herring, chicken liver, alcohol, ephedrine, pethidine. Because of these precautions the drug should only be used if no other form of treatment is appropriate.

Others

Isocarboxazid (Marplan), tranylcypromine (Parnate).

d. *Tryptophan (Optimax, Pacitron)*

L-tryptophan 2–6 G/day is used in some cases of depression.

e. Lithium *(Camcolit, Priadel, Liskonium)*

Lithium carbonate is effective in treating mania and is used increasingly to prevent relapse in manic-depressive psychosis. The drug is toxic producing drowsiness, tremor, ataxia, vomiting and diarrhoea. It is almost totally excreted by the kidney, and renal function should be assessed before starting the drug. Begin with a dose of 750–1500 mg a day and monitor blood level to achieve a steady state of 0.6–1.2 mmol/l plasma. This will take about 10 days. Thereafter blood should be checked every 4–8 weeks. In patients with an established history of manic depressive psychosis or recurrent depression and who can be relied upon to co-operate, this drug given indefinitely will significantly reduce the risk of relapse or readmission to hospital. However, reports of toxicity are frequent (e.g. renal damage with polyuria, thyroid suppression) and the drug administration should be supervised at an appropriate clinic.

Hypnotics and sedatives

These drugs are administered for the symptomatic relief of insomnia, agitation and panic.

a. Benzodiazepines (see p. 115)

Nitrazepam (Mogadon) 5–10 mg is a safe and reliable hypnotic for the treatment of insomnia. Flurazepam (Dalmane) and Temazepam (Normison) are others.

b. Barbiturates

Duration of action depends on stability of side-chain, tissue absorption and rate of kidney excretion. They are detoxicated in the liver.

Dangers: Addiction; suicidal attempts; skin sensitivity reactions. Barbiturates are best avoided in psychiatry where the duration of illness increases risk of habituation.

c. Chloral hydrate

Inexpensive and relatively safe. Gastric irritation is an occasional drawback.

Dose: 1–2 G

Also dichloralphenazone (Welldorm) as tablet or elixir (1–2, 650 mg tabs, 10–20 ml elixir).

d. Paraldehyde

A safe but unpleasant hypnotic: malodorous breath.

Dose: 2–10 ml orally or intramuscularly. Now used only in status epilepticus, delirium or severe mania. Must be given by a glass syringe.

e. Doriden (Glutethimide)

Said to be safe and relatively non-addictive. May cause nausea and skin rash.

Dose: 250–500 mg.

f. Morphine/Hyoscine

Valuable for acutely restless or violent case. Now rarely used.

Dose: Morphine sulphate 15 mg with hyoscine hydrobromide 0.6 mg.

FURTHER READING

Crammer J L, Barraclough B, Heine B M 1978 The use of drugs in psychiatry. Gaskell Books, London

24

Physical treatments

Physical treatments have developed rapidly in the last 50 years. Many were crude and empirical; some, like malarial therapy for cerebral syphilis and insulin coma therapy for schizophrenia, have been replaced by drugs; others, like electro-convulsive therapy and psychosurgery have been refined and have survived. The main developments in the last 20 years have been in psychopharmacology.

Electro-convulsive therapy (ECT)
Can be given to suitable patients in out-patient departments as well as in hospital.

Technique
1. Physical examination with special reference to chest and heart disease (chest X-ray and ECG if indicated).
2. Proper psychological preparation, giving patient clear account of the treatment and obtaining informed consent. Privacy before and during treatment and presence of familiar figures on recovery helpful.
3. No food or drink for at least five hours beforehand. Empty bowel and bladder. Remove dentures.
4. Atropine sulphate 0.6 mg 45-60 minutes before treatment or intravenously before anaesthetic.
5. Intravenous anaesthetic. Thiopentone (Pentothal) 0.25-0.5 G is slower than methohexitone and allows the patient to sleep longer in the early phases of recovery. A muscle relaxant — usually suxamethonium chloride (Scoline) about 50 mg — is injected through the same needle. Insufflation of oxygen given before convulsion and afterwards until respiration is restored. A mouth gag is inserted.
6. Convulsion is induced usually by a machine with automatic timing and a choice of wave forms. The stimulus is the minimum necessary to produce a generalised convulsion: usually of the order of 140 volts for 0.5 seconds. Saline pad electrodes are used. In bilateral ECT these are applied to the fronto-temporal areas. In unilateral ECT the electrodes are applied to the temple and the mastoid process on the same side (non-dominant).

Contraindications

Recent myocardial infarction or cerebrovascular accident, severe pulmonary disease. These are relative contraindications to be weighed against serious suicidal risk. Old age is not a contraindication.

Indications and effectiveness

The main indication is *severe depressive illness*. Symptoms predicting a good response to ECT include sudden onset and short duration, self reproach, retardation, weight loss, early waking and delusions. Unfavourable indicators are hypochondriasis and an hysterical personality.

In primary depressive illness severe enough to require admission ECT is at least as good as tricyclic antidepressants (and superior in females). An MRC trial (1965) showed the following recovery rates after four weeks: ECT 71 per cent, imipramine 52 per cent, phenelzine 30 per cent and placebo 39 per cent. ECT has the added advantage of speedier response compared with antidepressants.

ECT is less effective in mania and is inferior to drug treatment in schizophrenia, except when depressive symptoms are prominent.

Side effects

In the hours following treatment mild confusion and headache are common. If more than four treatments are given temporary memory impairment is frequent. It is rarely troublesome and recovers spontaneously over the next 3-4 weeks. There are no permanent memory effects. Unilateral treatment probably produces less memory impairment per treatment, but more treatments are usually necessary for a course to be effective.

Mortality

3-4/100 000 treatments and much lower than the mortality from suicide and other causes in untreated and drug treated depression.

Mechanism of action

Unknown. Various theories have suggested effects on protein synthesis and membrane permeability in the brain. Multiple ECT in rats leads to increased sensitivity of post-synoptic receptors to mono-amines, and ECT may thus potentiate the action of 5-H.T. and dopamine transmitter.

Functional neurosurgery

History

In the late 1940's thousands of patients were treated by standard leucotomy — a blind procedure by which the frontal white matter was divided with a blunt instrument through temporal burr-holes. The operation relieved anxiety, depressive and obsessional symptoms but often led to crippling after-effects, notably epilepsy and serious personality change, with severe apathy or disinhibition. It was virtually abandoned during the 1950's. In the last 25 years many modified procedures have been developed.

Anatomy

Emotional experience has been shown to be closely linked to the *limbic system,* comprising the hippocampus, amygdalum, fornix, the hippocampal and cingulate gyri, and the posterior part of the orbital frontal cortex. This system has complex connections with the frontal lobes, the hypothalamus and the brain stem. Current psychosurgery aims to produce limited lesions in the limbic system or its connections.

Techniques

    a. Undercutting of the medial third of the orbital cortex
    b. Bimedial leucotomy — aimed at the fronto-thalamic bundle
    c. Cingulectomy — anterior cingulate gyrus
    d. Stereotactic lesions. Many are being tested, e.g. lesions in the subcaudate nucleus, amygdala, thalamus and hypothalamus.
    All the above operations are bilateral.

Risks

Operative mortality is now negligible, and because of the limited lesions produced and stringent selection of patients, epilepsy and undesirable personality change are rare.

Indications

    a. Symptoms are a better guide than diagnosis. Tension, severe anxiety, chronic depression and obsessional symptoms respond best to surgery
    b. Operation is not carried out until other treatments have failed, but should not be unduly delayed
    c. Older patients improve more than the young
    d. In temporal lobe epilepsy (see p. 31) associated behavioural disturbance may be improved by surgery.

Results

In patients selected carefully the operations are successful in the majority of cases. At best there is complete symptomatic relief; even if this is not achieved the patient is able to benefit from rehabilitation and may respond to other treatments which had previously failed. These operations are probably too rarely done: less than five hundred in Britain annually.

FURTHER READING

Clare A 1979 Psychiatry in dissent: controversial issues in thought and practice. Tavistock, London

Kelly D 1976 Psychosurgery in the 1970's. British Journal of Hospital Medicine 16: 165-174

Royal College of Psychiatrists 1977 Memorandum on the use of ECT. British Journal of Psychiatry 131: 261-272

25

Psychiatric emergencies

Uncommon in general practice, frequent in casualty departments, psychiatric emergencies are worrying and time-consuming when they occur. In handling them a few general principles are crucial:

1. *Attitude.* However disturbed the behaviour of the patient, or those about him, behave calmly and quietly and seem confident and unhurried.

2. *Honesty.* Never lie to the patient or agree to any subterfuge relatives may suggest, e.g. pretending not to be a doctor, or that the patient is not being sent to a psychiatric hospital.

3. *History-taking.* The more disturbed the patient, the more helpful it is to take a short history from a relative or neighbour before seeing him.

4. *Use of force — compulsory admission.* Before using or advising physical restraint, the doctor should examine the patient, preferably alone. Most disturbed patients settle in a quiet atmosphere with a competent interviewer, but in the few cases where the patient's behaviour remains violent, uncooperative and an obvious danger to himself and others, there should be no delay in giving needed treatment, usually sedation prior to compulsory admission to hospital. If restraint is needed, a more than adequate number of assistants should be used, to reduce the risk of injury on both sides. Half measures are worse than useless.

Some common emergencies

Acute stress reactions
Panic, weeping, 'hysterics' and other signs of distress are often seen after personal or social disasters such as bereavements and bombings. They are quickly relieved by a period of sleep achieved by adequate sedation, e.g. diazepam 10 mg, chlordiazepoxide 20 mg or amylobarbitone sod. 200–400 mg orally. Such psychiatric casualties must be envisaged in all major disaster plans. Adequate treatment diminishes subsequent post-traumatic neurosis, and if not available interferes with the treatment of other victims.

Acute agitation

Agitation may be seen in phobic and anxiety states and in depressive illness. Severe neurotic emergencies are best managed by a single large oral or parenteral dose of a barbiturate, or a benzodiazepine. In agitated depression chlorpromazine 50 mg intramuscularly is often effective.

Paranoid delusions

Delusions of persecution may be the presenting symptom in schizophrenia, depression or senile psychoses. The patient may lock himself in his house to protect himself against his persecutors and entry may have to be forced with the help of relatives or the police. The patient may then agree to come to hospital although he may not admit that he is ill. In these suspicious patients a blunt, frank and honest approach is usually rewarded.

Alcohol and drugs

The noisy drunk may require the presence of the police for co-operation. An emetic may be used to hasten sobriety: drugs should be avoided. Always remember that drunkenness may conceal physical and psychiatric illness; head injury, depression and parasuicide are examples.

In incipient delirium tremens, start Vitamin B complex by injection, and give chlordiazepoxide 20–40 mg orally or by injection four-hourly.

Drug abuse may present with the 'bad trip' of the L.S.D. taker, the drunken gait and speech of the barbiturate taker, or the flushed hyperactivity of the amphetamine abuser. Phenothiazines should be given for L.S.D. reactions, and appropriate treatment for the others as necessary.

The drug addict taking heroin, opiates, etc. is usually young, aggressive, demanding, untruthful and persistent in his demands for supplies. He is usually knowledgeable about his condition and legal rights. If he claims to be a registered addict this should be checked with the Home Office who keep registers and provide a telephone service. Only methadone should be given, in a single dose of 5 to 10 mg seen to be taken, and the patient should then be referred to the nearest official clinic for addicts.

Suicidal attempts

Medical or surgical treatment of the emergency obviously takes precedence, but information about the circumstances should be collected at the time — it may be concealed or difficult to obtain later.

On recovery the depressed patient often feels better temporarily, or may conceal his persistent suicidal thoughts. All parasuicides should have a psychiatric examination.

The violent and hostile patient

Violence is surprisingly rare but may occur in acute mania, catatonic excitement, paranoid schizophrenia, some acute organic states, and in epileptic furor. Restraint, sedation and compulsory admission will usually be needed. The best emergency sedative in such cases is an injection of chlorpromazine 50 to 100 mg given through the clothing if need be. Morphine may be substituted if chlorpromazine is not available. In organic confusion, especially in epilepsy and in the elderly, paraldehyde 5 to 10 ml intramuscularly is effective and safe but smelly. For the noisy drunk apomorphine 5 to 8 mg is effective.

Hypomanic patients who are insightless and overcheerful may be irritable and hostile for short periods, especially when admission is suggested. Given time and patience they can usually be coaxed into co-operation. This is rarely feasible in acute schizophrenic and organic states, where if treatment is urgently indicated there should be no hesitation in ensuring that it is obtained, if necessary by compulsory admission.

FURTHER READING

Edwards J G 1976 Psychiatric aspects of civilian disasters. British Medical Journal 1: 944-947

26

Rehabilitation

Over the past thirty years there has been a gradual move from treatment in mental hospitals towards treatment at home, in out-patient clinics, day hospitals and the psychiatric units of general hospitals. However, predictions made twenty years ago of the rapid reduction or disappearance of mental hospitals have not proved correct. Psychiatric hospitals still house large numbers of patients suffering from chronic schizophrenia and for these and other patients programmes of social and occupational rehabilitation are essential.

For the rehabilitation of psychiatric patients the creation of a 'treatment team' is necessary. Psychiatrist, nurse, social worker, psychologist, occupational therapist and, to a smaller extent, physiotherapist and speech therapist will all have a part to play. Many psychiatric hospitals have developed the idea of a 'therapeutic community' in which all members of staff and patients meet regularly to discuss day-to-day problems and to help patients with their social difficulties. Programmes of work for patients help to restore confidence and to create a more realistic pattern of daily living. Most psychiatric hospitals now have industrial therapy departments, run by occupational therapists and nurses, where patients work regular hours for some financial reward. Patients whose work performance improves will often be referred to an industrial rehabilitation unit (run by the Department of Employment and Productivity) where the patient's working capacity is assessed and his ability to return to normal employment can be demonstrated.

In addition to social and occupational programmes for in-patients most mental health services now have a proportion of day patients. Patients suffering from chronic mental illness are encouraged to leave hospital and to return by day. Patients normally return to their own homes but where there is no suitable home, lodgings or a hostel provided by the local authority are used. The administration of long-acting phenothiazine drugs (see p. 114) to chronic schizophrenic patients has increased the number able to live outwith hospital. Despite these developments some patients with chronic disabilities, often multiple, e.g. schizophrenia, head injury, epilepsy, physical handicap, still require long-term care in hospital — the 'new long stay' patients.

The Mental Health Acts gave local authorities responsibility for providing services for the mentally ill living in the community. Most local authorities provided some social work or nursing services but few provided residential or day care.

The Social Work Acts extended this responsibility for community mental health services and there has been some increased provision of community services for the mentally ill by social work departments. However, such developments have been slow and the psychiatric services continue to provide the major part of the mental health service. In some places hospital annexes or hostels run jointly by the health service, social work department or by voluntary agencies have been developed. The contribution of social work to rehabilitation is of considerable importance. The social worker is trained to assess the social and family problems of the patient and to give advice about the services available to help. Social workers are also trained to help with the emotional problems of patients and their families and there should be constant co-operation between the social worker and the doctor.

A progressive mental health service which has created a 'team approach' to psychiatric care in the community and emergency domiciliary care ('Crisis Intervention') will often lead to a reduction in admission rates and bed requirements.

FURTHER READING

Royal College of Psychiatrists 1980 Psychiatric rehabilitation in the 1980s.

Further reading

The student of psychiatry is well served with review articles and paperbacks on special areas; most of the further reading suggested at the end of chapters is readily available and a selection should be made according to interest and the recommendation of teachers. All in turn suggest further reading and will serve as an introduction to the specialist literature.

Many short general text books are available. We recommend:

Clare A 1980 Psychiatry in dissent. Tavistock, London: a readable book on controversial issues

Merskey H, Tonge W L 1974 Psychiatric illness. Bailliere, Tindal and Cox, London: which deals capably with minor psychiatry and the elements of psychotherapy

In clinical work and for reference the following larger texts should be consulted:

Forrest A D 1979 Companion to psychiatric studies. Churchill Livingstone, Edinburgh

Granville-Grossman K 1971, 1976, 1979 Recent advances in clinical psychiatry, 3 volumes. Churchill Livingstone, Edinburgh

Hill P, Murray R, Thorley A 1979 Essentials of postgraduate psychiatry. Academic Press, London

Sim M 1974 Guide to psychiatry. Churchill Livingstone, Edinburgh

For the main specialities:

Brown D, Pedder J 1979 Introduction to psychotherapy. Tavistock Publications, London

Lishman W A 1978 Organic psychiatry. BSP, London

Mowbray R M 1979 Psychology in relation to medicine. Churchill Livingstone, Edinburgh

Rutter M 1979 Child psychiatry: modern approaches. BSP, London

Craft M (ed) 1979 Tredgold's mental retardation. Bailliere Tindall, London

Glossary

Some of the terms used in these notes may be unfamiliar to students or used in an unfamiliar sense. The following explanations indicate how the terms are used in the notes and are not strict definitions. Definitions of other technical words and phrases can be traced by using the index.

Abstract thinking. The ability to use concepts and ideas independently of concrete objects.

Acalculia. Loss of the ability to calculate.

Affect. Mood, feeling or emotion.

Agraphia. Loss of the ability to write.

Alexia. Loss of the ability to read.

Anterograde amnesia. Inability to remember events occurring *after* a brain injury, even though the patient was apparently conscious (cf. retrograde amnesia).

Aphasia (dysphasia). Loss or partial loss of the ability to use language (i.e. to speak or to recognise the spoken word).

Asthenic build. Tall slender body-shape (cf. pyknic).

Autistic thinking. Thinking which is unduly self-directed.

Confabulation. False recall associated with failure in memory.

Constitution. The total hereditary characteristics of a person.

Conversion. The mechanism whereby anxiety is transformed into a physical symptom.

Compulsion. An impulse to carry out or repeat certain actions resisted by the patient and usually recognised by him as meaningless.

Curator Bonis. A person appointed by the Courts in Scotland to look after a patient's affairs when he is incapable of doing so himself or of directing others to do so.

Delirium. Transitory or potentially reversible mental confusion.

Delusions. False beliefs or attitudes with no basis in reality, often illogical.

Dementia. The end-stage of intellectual deterioration. An irreversible state of brain damage.

Depersonalisation. A feeling that one has lost one's feelings or identity or that one is unreal.

Derealisation. A feeling that things in the environment are no longer real.

Dereistic thinking. Thinking concerned with phantastic or imaginary events.

Dissociation. A process whereby certain psychological activities lose their relationship to the remainder of the personality and function more or less independently.

Dysarthria. Faulty articulation of speech

Dysmnesia. Partial disturbance of memory (cf. amnesia).

Echopraxia. Automatic and purposeless imitation of another person's movements.

Euphoria. Mood of well-being, sometimes inappropriate (e.g. in presence of physical illness).

Extraversion. The general characteristic of those individuals whose interests and reactions are directed outwards (cf. introversion where interests are predominantly directed inwards).

Fetishism. Condition in which sexual excitement is aroused by the presence of a non-sexual object.

Hallucination. Convincing perception in any sensory modality (e.g. vision, hearing, taste, smell, touch) independent of the relevant stimulation (cf. illusion).

Hypochondriasis. Morbid concern with health or with bodily processes.

Illusion. Mistaken perception in any sensory modality (cf. hallucination).

Incidence. The number of cases of an illness which arise in a population in a given period (cf. prevalence).

Integration of personality. The extent to which an individual's personal qualities are unified or consistent.

Knight's move thinking. Reasoning which omits an essential step.

Libido. Sexual drive or urg'

Neologism. A specially coined or nonsensical word (e.g. 'brillig').

Neurasthenia. Term applied to neurotic disorder characterised by weakness and fatiguability.

Neuroticism. The tendency or predisposition of an individual to become neurotic.

Obsession. A dominating and repetitive experience or idea which cannot be resisted even although recognised as senseless.

Oedipal situation. Freud's explanation, based on the story of King Oedipus, of the emotional indentifications within the family. The son identified with father has strong emotional ties with mother.

Orientation. Knowledge of one's identity and one's situation in place and time and in regard to other persons.

Paranoid. Literally, false reasoning. Having delusions, usually of persecution. *Paranoid personality* — an individual who is suspicious and sensitive.

Perseveration. Persistence or recurrence of an idea or action. Inability to shift from one task to another.

Personality. All the unique personal qualities of an individual.

Phantasticant. Drug which produces phantastic experiences, such as visual hallucinations, in normal individuals.

Placebo. From Latin 'I will please'. An inert tablet or liquid which produces relief of symptoms. Used in drug trials to compare effect of new drug with improvement produced by patients response to the 'dummy' preparation.

Prevalence. The amount of an illness which exists in a population at a particular time (cf. incidence).

Psychiatric social worker. A specially trained social worker who is responsible for investigating and remedying the patient's social, family and occupational circumstances.

Psychodynamics. The study of the way in which past experiences and attitudes produce present symptoms.

Psychopathology. The study of the ideas and experiences which occur in psychological disorders.

Pyknic build. Short thick-set body shape (cf. asthenic).

Rapport. Mutually confident relationship between two people (e.g. patient and doctor).

Retrograde amnesia. Inability to remember events occurring *prior to* a brain injury or to brain damage due to an acute illness (cf. anterograde amnesia).

Sado-masochism. Sexual gratification aroused by inflicting pain (sadism) or suffering pain (masochism).

Siblings. Children of the same parents.

Stereotyped act. A uniform, persistent and repetitive sequence of behaviour, usually having no purpose.

Transvestism. Condition in which sexual gratification is obtained from wearing clothing of the opposite sex.

Volition. The act of deciding upon and initiating a course of action.

Index